Shared Struggles

Ann F. Schrooten • Barry P. Markovitz

Shared Struggles

Stories from Parents and Pediatricians Caring for Children with Serious Illnesses

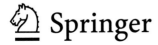 Springer

Ann F. Schrooten
Chandler, AZ
USA

Barry P. Markovitz
Anesthesiology Critical Care Medicine
USC Keck School of Medicine and
Children's Hospital Los Angeles
Los Angeles, CA
USA

ISBN 978-3-030-68019-0   ISBN 978-3-030-68020-6   (eBook)
https://doi.org/10.1007/978-3-030-68020-6

This Copernicus imprint is published by the registered company Springer Nature Switzerland AG
The registered company address is: Gewerbestrasse 11, 6330 Cham, Switzerland

Dedicated to Jack. May his memory always be a blessing.

Foreword

My mentor in palliative care fellowship once told me that most of what we do as palliative care providers can be summed up as helping the hospital learn and understand what is going on in the patient's room. By "the hospital" he meant the whole panoply of medical and psychosocial care providers assigned to the patient, orbiting near and far from the bedside, anybody who might open up one of our consult notes to read the documentation of conversations in which we asked parents to tell us about their hopes and worries, about the sources of their strength and support, and most importantly, about who their child is, not as a patient, but as a person, because a parent's portrait of a child is a portrait of a parent's values and a family's values. By "the room" he meant not just the space enclosed by the four brightly colored walls, but the emotional and spiritual milieu in which the patient and family lived, loved, and hoped—the ordinary physical space being a metonymy for an extraordinary metaphysical space that housed not just the bodies of a patient and their family, but also their stories and their spirits.

This book is an exquisite collection of just that kind of story. To read it is to learn just how much goes on inside "the room," just how rich and terrifying and beautiful any one family's experience of the hospital can be, how totally different every family is in their unique phenotype of daily struggle and triumph, how very much the same they are in the example of profound loving they make to us all.

But this book collects the story of what is going on in another room, one that intersects and overlaps with the physical and metaphysical spaces of the patient's room. The doctor's room is a workroom on the unit, but also the empty storeroom into which they might retreat to collect their thoughts and feelings, or the car in which they make their commute, and like the patient's room, the doctor's room expands to encompass their home, their own family, their friends. It is the headspace and the heart-space in which they attend to the patients and families under their care.

To collect and juxtapose these stories is already to make something beautiful for the world at large and useful for the community of care for children with serious illnesses and their families. But *Shared Struggles* takes the risk of committing itself to reconciling these stories, by means of parent and physician commentary which engage with the content from positions of equal and complimentary expertise. That risk elevates the beauty and use of the book such that it becomes something entirely astonishing and necessary and completely one-of-a-kind: a textbook of connection between physician and patient and family, one that illustrates in real time the process of reconciliation between the lived experience of each party, a reconciliation that is the fundamental act of pediatric medicine.

As pediatric medical providers, we talk about the art of medicine as something we practice upon patients, not often recognizing that patients and families, and parents especially, practice their own art of medicine, not on their children or themselves, but upon us. They are called to manage us, in the course of their child's illness, just as much as we are called to manage their children, as they partner with us in loving care, seeking always to find a way to accept the help we offer while protecting their child from any harm we might do. You cannot tell someone how to practice such an art any more than you can tell them how to be compassionate, or empathetic, or kind. But that does not mean instruction is impossible. Such attributes, and such art, can be fostered and encouraged into sturdy practice. You cannot simply tell someone how to make a genuine connection with their patient, how to shape their professional boundaries, not as lines in the sand, but as contours along the heart. You cannot just tell someone how to balance advocacy for their child with trust for a provider, how to put faith in the love of a stranger for their child and never lose faith with oneself. But you can certainly show them how to do it, as this collection shows us, with unparalleled richness and sincerity, over and over again.

Christopher Adrian
Clinical Assistant Professor of Pediatrics, USC Keck School of Medicine and
Attending Physician, Division of Comfort and Palliative Care Medicine
Department of Anesthesiology Critical Care Medicine,
Children's Hospital Los Angeles
Los Angeles, CA
USA

Acknowledgments

When the idea of what we wanted this book to look like was solidified, we knew the people we needed to make it happen – the parents of medically complex children and the pediatricians caring for these children – were exceptionally busy people. Asking parents deep in the trenches of caring for their child and physicians overwhelmed with patient and academic responsibilities to take the time to write a story for this book was, admittedly, an intimidating endeavor. We reached out to our respective networks of parents and colleagues not knowing what to expect, but hoping for the best. The response we received was overwhelmingly kind and supportive. As the book took shape and the areas we wanted to focus on became clearer, we were limited in the number of stories we could include. As a result, we were unable to include all of the stories we received. The contributors listed are those whose stories are included in the book; however, every story that was contributed was instrumental in the making of the book. Every person who contributed a story validated the importance of the book and every story and lesson shared was carried with us as we wrote our commentaries. Thank you to each and every person who contributed a story for giving your time, your heart, and your insight to make this book the unique and valuable resource it is.

Thank you also to the people who graciously gave their time to review drafts, provide feedback and edits, and supported us throughout the process from beginning to end, especially Bridget, Kathie, Jenni, and Erin.

Finally, thank you Jack for being the thread that connected us. You are a beautiful soul who taught us all so much without ever speaking a word.

Parent Contributors

Cynthia Bissell; Angela Capello; Sarah E. Dunn; Regina Gort; Ann Gramuglia; Stephanie Hogan; Christy Holton; Erin Killen; Allison Lefebvre; Shannon K. Mashinchi; Brian McCullagh;
Jennifer Reming; Sara Scaparotti; Rei Schenk; Ann F. Schrooten; Jennifer Shaffer; Kristin Skenderi; Diane Smith-Hoban; Mary Beth Sutter; Erin Ward

Physician Contributors

Wendy P. Bernatavicius, MD; Jay Berry, MD MPH, Harman Chawla, MD;
Paul A. Checchia, MD; Sabrina F. Derrington, MD; Robert J. Graham, MD;
Jack Green, MD; Zena Leah Harris, MD; Daniel D. Im, MD;
Kelly N. Michelson, MD MPH; Sholeen T. Nett, MD PhD; Katie R. Nielsen, MD MPH;
Lauren Rissman, MD; Nathan S. Rosenberg, MD; Amy RL Rule, MD MPH;
Pamela M. Schuler, MD; Tressia M. Shaw, MD; Steven M. Smith, MD;
Kellie C. Snooks, MD; Jaime Twanow, MD; Amy E. Vinson, MD;
Elisha D. Waldman, MD; Sally L. Davidson Ward, MD MPH; Pedro
Weisleder, MD PhD

Contents

Part I Compassion

1 What Matters at the End 3

2 I Did Not Have to Fix It 9

3 No Wrong Decisions 13

4 Reuniting Families 19

5 Leading with Compassion 23

6 Minute by Minute, Step by Step 27

7 Seek Permission First 31

8 A Sacred Relationship 35

9 Kids Like These 39

10 A Smile Worth Saving 43

Part II Trust

11 Team Harlie 51

12 Best Laid Plans 57

13 If We Are Paying Attention 61

14 Full Disclosure 67

15 The Photograph 73

16 Learning Together 77

17 Altered Path 83

18 The Befores and the Afters 87

19 Not Everyone Is Born a Superhero 91

20 Beyond the Numbers 95

21   Shared Experience 101

22   Tying the Thread into a Bond 105

Part III   Communication

23   A Voice That Doesn't Use Words 113

24   Brave the Difficult Conversation 119

25   A Roadmap 123

26   Teamwork 129

27   Relearning to Listen 135

28   Words Matter 141

29   Trust Their Voice 147

30   Knowing Your Family 151

31   Advocacy Is Not Anger 157

32   Where Is the Doctor? 161

33   Failure to Communicate 167

34   When a Patient and Family Forever Change Your World 173

35   Respect: A Two-Way Street 181

Part IV   Hope

36   Persistence of Hope: A Story in Two Acts 189

37   Can I Offer You Advice? 195

38   The Life of the Party 201

39   Every Single Second Worth It 209

40   Partners in Hope 217

41   Answers for Rosie 223

42   We Treat Souls, Not Just Bodies 227

43   Never Give Up 231

44   The Sliver of Sky 237

45   The Many Voices of Hope 243

46   Mothers Club 249

Glossary 255

Index 257

About the Editors

Ann F. Schrooten and her husband, Mark, are parents of four children. Their son, Jack, was born with a rare congenital muscular dystrophy that affected his muscles, eyes, and brain. Jack required the support of a ventilator to help him breathe; he was non-verbal, non-mobile, and required round-the-clock care. Yet, despite all his challenges, Jack woke up every morning with a smile on his face and eyes that sparkled with the anticipation of a new day. Jack lived a love-filled life until his death at the age of 15. Ann has experienced hundreds of encounters with doctors and other medical professionals, beginning with Jack's premature birth and complicated first year where he spent many months in the Pediatric Intensive Care Unit, through his diagnosis odyssey, the many procedures, surgeries, and hospitalizations he endured, his transition to palliative care and, finally, to hospice care at the end of his life. Because of Jack, Ann has connected with a large network of other parents of medically complex children from across the country and the globe. She is the founder of The Willow Tree Foundation, an Arizona non-profit organization that funds respite for parents of medically fragile children (http://willowtreefoundation.org). She also created TouchStones of Compassionate Care®, a program that promotes compassion in the delivery of healthcare. (www.touchstonesofcc.blogspot.com). She lives in Chandler, Arizona, and enjoys writing, kayaking, and hiking.

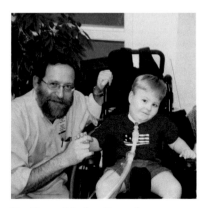

Dr. Barry Markovitz and Jack Schrooten

Barry P. Markovitz earned his Bachelor of Science degree at Washington & Jefferson College in Washington, Pennsylvania, and his medical degree at the University of Pennsylvania. He completed his pediatric residency at Children's Memorial Hospital in Chicago (now Ann & Robert H. Lurie Children's Hospital of Chicago) and a residency in anesthesiology at the Hospital of the University of Pennsylvania. Following his fellowship in pediatric anesthesiology and critical care medicine at the Children's Hospital of Philadelphia, he then joined the faculty at Washington University School of

Medicine in 1990 and was an attending pediatric anesthesiologist and intensivist at St. Louis Children's Hospital. He moved in 2006 to become the director of critical care medicine and medical director of the PICU at Children's Hospital Los Angeles (CHLA) and is a professor of clinical pediatrics and anesthesiology at the University of Southern California Keck School of Medicine. In 2018, he became the chair of the Department of Anesthesiology Critical Care Medicine at CHLA.

He has a strong interest in medical informatics and has been the editor of PedsCCM: The Web Site for Pediatric Critical Care Medicine (http://PedsCCM. org/) since its inception in 1995. He was a co-founding member of the Virtual PICU and was the chair of the scientific review committee of VPS, LLC. His interest in evidence-based medicine and clinical epidemiology involves editing the Evidence-Based Journal Club on the PedsCCM website (nearly 1000 evidence-based reviews of literature in critical care) and completing a master's degree in public health at St. Louis University School of Public Health in 2003. He has been involved in the planning and/or conducting of numerous multicenter trials in pediatric critical care medicine and recently completed a term as the chair of the Scientific Steering Committee of the PALISI (Pediatric Acute Lung Injury and Sepsis Investigators; http://palisi. org) research network. He has authored or co-authored over 70 peer-reviewed publications, chapters, and monographs and given over 80 public presentations and lectures. Barry and his wife, Martha, have been married for 35 years and have two adult daughters. He lives in Los Angeles, California, and enjoys running, hiking, and reading fictionalized history books.

Ann and Barry met more than 20 years ago when Barry was one of the intensivists who cared for Ann's son, Jack, in the Pediatric Intensive Care Unit where he spent much of the first year of his life. Ann will always remember the first time she met Barry. It was early one morning in the PICU; she was sitting in a chair next to Jack's bed when he came over to talk to her about Jack. What she remembers is not what he said, but what he did. Before he said anything, he gently knelt down by the chair so that he was eye level with her rather than looking down on her when he spoke. This simple act was so impactful because it was the exception, not the norm. To most, this may seem like a meaningless, trivial gesture. On the contrary, Ann will tell you that it is indicative of the special person and doctor Barry is – he is humble, he is respectful, and he is kind. Four months after that first encounter, Barry would show up at Jack's bedside and offer to do something that was, again, the exception, not the norm.

When Jack was discharged from the PICU needing the support of a home ventilator, Barry offered to take on the unconventional role of managing Jack's care. The expectation was that Jack would only need the support of the ventilator for a short time and would quickly wean from it. After several years, when it was clear that Jack would need long-term ventilatory support, his care was taken over by a pediatric pulmonologist who specialized in the management of ventilator-dependent children. However, despite this "break" in the doctor-patient relationship, Ann and Barry stayed in touch over the course of Jack's life – Ann always seeking out Barry's advice and reason in connection with Jack's care, and Barry always willing to listen and help in any way that he could.

Barry's recollection of Jack and Ann in the early days did not seem particularly extraordinary. Jack was a patient and Ann was his mother. The lessons that Barry learned from them were simple and only later became generalizable. Ann knew Jack better than anyone. She paid attention to detail and could always be trusted to be Jack's best advocate. No one else on the healthcare team could do what she did. So Barry got "trained" early by Jack and Ann to listen to them – carefully – respect their concerns and address them. And even if there was not an immediate answer, he paid attention. Barry also learned that a diagnosis and a prognosis are, at best, educated guesses. Every patient is different and even with the same specific genetic mutation, each may manifest a condition differently. Finally, he learned that the often-vaulted "quality of life" – like beauty – is in the eye of the beholder. The only beholders that matter in this area are the patient and the parent.

Shortly after Jack's death, Barry pitched the idea of this book to Ann – who jumped on board without hesitation, eager to fill the void of Jack's absence and the unfamiliar free time she now had. This book was written and compiled over the course of 5 years, but its roots were planted over 20 years ago in a Pediatric Intensive Care Unit when a special connection was made between a little boy named Jack, his mom, and a doctor who agreed to follow a kid on a vent even though it was outside the box. While they never imagined where that connection would take them, it seems only fitting that it would lead to the unconventional bringing together of parents and doctors to share their personal stories and experiences in this first-of-its-kind book. They have learned a lot from each other over the years and are grateful for the opportunity to continue the conversation through this book and the honest and heartfelt stories told by both sides of the physician-patient/parent relationship.

Introduction

Respectful communication is really valued by parents of medically complex kids. Invite me into the dialogue and ask my opinion, or at the very least, respect my concerns. In our world, we have been forced to become experts in a field we did not choose.... I can see how a resident neurosurgeon wants to feel some respect for their years of grueling work to get where they are. But so do I.

–Parent

That moment of contact, of connection and real communication with this *person*, remains a pivotal moment in my career.... I always take care now to allow for space for children to express their voice, in whatever form that might take. To not expect that communication occur on my terms, but rather to be open to whatever terms and means of communication, no matter how subtle, a child might choose.

–Physician

There are approximately three million children in the United States living with complex medical conditions. With advances in medicine, this number will only grow as children born with rare and life-limiting conditions live longer. Children with medical complexity have chronic health problems that affect multiple organ systems and result in functional limitations, high healthcare needs, and often require the use of medical technology. The parents of these children become experts in their child's condition. They connect with other parents; they travel to world-renowned Children's Hospitals for second and third opinions; they ask questions; and they are relentless advocates for their children. In emergency rooms, ICUs, hospital rooms, and clinics, these parents spend a lot of time with the healthcare team and often interact with as many as ten or more pediatric subspecialists caring for their child. These interactions can often be filled with tension, misunderstanding, and conflict. Parents make assumptions about physicians (e.g., "He doesn't care." "She thinks I'm being difficult."), and physicians make assumptions about parents (e.g., "They don't understand their child's disease." "She's an angry mom."). On the other hand, there are also many instances of great compassion and understanding, and encounters where parents and physicians are deeply affected and changed by their interactions and relationships.

We know that stories are one of the most fundamental and effective ways to engage and teach our fellow human beings. This is the first book to share stories from both sides of the physician-patient/parent experience through richly detailed and heartfelt stories contributed by parents of medically complex children with a wide range of disorders and diseases, and by pediatricians practicing in the many subspecialties that provide care to these children.

The parent stories are contributed by parents from across the United States. Each story emotionally describes an encounter or relationship with a physician that had a significant impact on the parent and their child. The parent stories share compassionate and positive physician interactions, as well as instances where their child's physician let them and their child down. To maintain anonymity, the physicians and hospitals involved are not identified by name and some parents have chosen not to use their child's real name. The physician stories are contributed by physicians practicing at many of the best Children's Hospitals throughout the country. These stories poignantly tell of encounters and relationships physicians had with their patients and parents that significantly impacted them and served as learning moments in their career. In those stories where the family's consent was not obtained, the names of patients and parents have been changed to protect privacy and patients have been de-identified. To further protect privacy, the parent and physician contributors are not identified with their stories.

Following each story are commentaries written by the editors; a parent commentary written by Ann, and a physician commentary written by Barry. The commentaries provide an independent perspective on the events and messages conveyed by the story contributor and are intended to encourage reflection, inquiry, and discussion. We understand and respect that we cannot truly put ourselves into the shoes of the storyteller, we can only draw upon our own experiences when sharing our perspectives and "take-aways" from each story. With respect to the physician commentaries – I (Barry) want to add that a time honored tradition in the medical profession is to not throw your colleagues under the bus. Perhaps too honored. Some of my commentaries may verge on a criticism of my unknown colleagues. I do not pretend to put myself in their place, as I cannot even fathom all the intricacies of issues they were dealing with at the time. And we have only one side of the story in most cases. However, as with possession and the law, perception is 9/10ths of reality. If these parents perceived a lack of empathy or proper communication on the part of physicians, that was their reality. Only now do we have the hindsight of the "retrospectoscope" – the ability to look backwards in time and suggest a different course.

We learn and change most from hearing stories that strike a chord with us. The parent and physician stories are grouped under four parts that touch on the universal themes of compassion, trust, communication, and hope, and will strike a chord with everyone who is on the giving and receiving side of healthcare. By giving a voice to both parents and physicians, and by listening and learning from their stories, we hope this book can be a bridge to better understanding between the parent expert and the medical expert and lead to improved communication, minimize conflicts, and foster trust and compassion among physicians, patients, and families. A strong partnership between the parent and the physician is vital to ensuring the best care possible for this unique and growing population of children.

> Could a greater miracle take place than for us to look through each other's eyes for an instant?
>
> *–Henry David Thoreau*

Part I

Compassion

Compassion is not a virtue. It is a commitment. It's not something we have or don't have. It's something we choose to practice. –Brené Brown

What Matters at the End

1

Summer was at its peak and so was the heat. Our beloved dog had just died and my husband and I were trying to distract ourselves by going for a walk in the neighborhood park. The familiar plethora of summer smells was filling the air—freshly cut grass, an early dinner cooking on a nearby grill, and the many hard-to-classify odors that come on waves of hot air in late July. I understand how morbid, strange, and even irresponsible it sounds, but it took the death of our dog to open my eyes to our son's suffering. I knew our youngest son was going to die. I had known for 2 years that due to faulty genes passed down by me and my husband, toxins were accumulating in his little body, progressively destroying his nervous system and spinal cord. We watched the disease ruthlessly claim his ability to sit, smile, see, and eat. With each reversed milestone, we became increasingly aware of the trajectory of his illness and intimately familiar with both his and our own suffering. Yet, the human heart has an amazing capacity to adjust and adapt and 2 years after the diagnosis, trained as it was to suffering, my heart had grown numb. I believe it took the death of our dog to crack it open again.

Two years prior, a few months after receiving Joey's diagnosis, we made the decision to have a gastrostomy tube (G-tube) placed into his stomach to give direct access for supplemental feeding, hydration, and medication. At that point, he was still nursing and able to eat pureed foods by mouth; yet, our medical team mindlessly followed the standard protocol of scheduling a consultation with a GI specialist, undoubtedly because our son's diagnosis included words such as "genetic," "degenerative," and "neurological." During the initial consultation, the GI specialist did a beautiful job explaining why Joey needed a G-tube, referencing risks of aspiration pneumonia, dehydration, and issues with administering medication. Her arguments in favor of a G-tube were presented as fact. Never once did she ask if a G-tube indeed was in line with our philosophy of care, nor did she mention what the alternative (no intervention) might look like. A couple of months later, during the preoperative huddle, we had another extensive conversation, this time with the surgical team regarding the risks and concerns around general anesthesia administered to a child with decreased neuromuscular function. No one, however, told us that

© Springer Nature Switzerland AG 2021
A. F. Schrooten, B. P. Markovitz, *Shared Struggles,*
https://doi.org/10.1007/978-3-030-68020-6_1

providing feeding and hydration through artificial means would likely extend life, that it could prolong the natural process of dying, and contrary to our goal of keeping Joey comfortable, could also add to his suffering. These were things we were left to learn through first-hand experience.

Back from our walk, guided by our hearts as opposed to an anticipated medical event, my husband and I realized we did not know the protocol—when to call or how to communicate to Joey's medical team that the end was near. There was no medical emergency, we did not "need" them for anything, but we chose to reach out because we wanted them there.

Joey's pulmonologist answered our call late on a Saturday afternoon in July. It was a short conversation. My husband informed him of how Joey had reached a new level of decline and that we were going to discontinue his feeds with the anticipation that he would pass in the next several days. My husband did not say that our hearts could no longer bear the pain of watching our son suffer, that keeping him alive by providing his frail little body with nutrition and his lungs with oxygen felt selfish and unkind, yet somehow the message still translated the same. Less than 24 hours later, on his way home from a family event, John walked through our front door. No white coat, no stethoscope, no hand sanitizer, or pulse oximeter in tow. He simply showed up as another guest in a house full of love-filled mourners.

By this point, we had long ruled out a miracle and any potential solution to the unfixable problem that a fatal diagnosis is. Instead, connection and the presence of others became the most vital and valuable gifts to us. Connection takes us deeper than job descriptions, titles, and formalities, but it needs to take its own shape and can never be forced or fabricated. It is comforting because of its authenticity. It cannot be achieved through a formula or a prescribed set of best practices; it can be as simple and profound as a pediatric pulmonologist, in civilian clothing, sitting on a couch with a glass of wine and his dying patient gently cradled in his arms.

Joey went 14 days without food and 10 days without water. Against all our parental instincts, yet fueled by pure, deep, and unconditional love for our son, not the opinions of our medical team, we were able to push our own needs aside and allow for what needed to happen. We simply had no clue how gruesome and drawn out death can be. Predictions around the number of days or hours he had left to live varied by the day and the conviction of the person assessing him. In hindsight, I would say those predictions are both empty and inconsequential. It is nearly impossible to predict the final breath. However, 14 days without sustenance both looked and felt like the definition of starvation, which was the opposite of what we hoped and prayed for. Two years of listening to the rattling in Joey's little chest and the sound of secretions pooling in the back of his throat led us to believe he would die of pneumonia—that it would be "quick" and "peaceful." We were wrong on both accounts.

Friday, August 11, 2017—a day etched on my mind and soul and likely in every cell and muscle fiber of my body, forever. The unforgiving August sun made our house feel small, airless, and muggy, causing me to pity the large number of friends, family, and members of Joey's care team who were struggling to get comfortable in our tiny living room.

After listening to our lamentations about a seemingly endless ending, and perhaps in an attempt to protect our hearts and minds, Joey's neurologist reluctantly said, "Death isn't always peaceful. The final moments can be rather traumatic for the ones having to watch their loved one die." He went on to explain how air hunger and terminal agitation appear agonizing, but are not uncomfortable for the dying child. His full-of-compassion-non-sugar-coated-hard-to-hear truth turned out to be a prophetic and considerate warning of our son's final hour.

The end itself was as sacred as it was excruciating. At 3:27 a.m. the following morning, our friends Scott and Susie, who had offered to take the night shift so Sam and I could get some sleep, let us know Joey's breathing had changed and that we should probably come and get him. When Sam brought him into our bedroom, Joey appeared to be in deep distress, frequently gasping for air as his face gradually changed color. For 10 minutes we watched as our son's body shut down until eventually the breathing stopped all together and he died, not so peacefully, in my husband's arms.

There is nothing more basic to parenting than to feed your child, and there is nothing more painful than mercifully denying your child sustenance. Even though Joey was unable to eat by mouth the last 18 months of his life, my desire to nurture him never subsided. The various combinations of oats, quinoa, avocado, veggies, fruit, peanut butter, prunes, coconut oil, beets, and apple sauce I ran through our Vitamix blender every day undeniably made some part of me feel better, but I think it benefitted him as well. And no, we did not agree to our son's G-tube surgery because we had to or were forced to, no one is. We did it because it felt like the right thing to do. Joey never learned to drink out of a bottle and, as a result, dehydration and, eventually hunger, did indeed make him and everyone around him miserable.

Our decision to provide nutrition through a G-tube unquestionably brought comfort and improved everyone's quality of life, but a conversation about the end and what it could look like would have prepared us and saved us from unnecessary self-doubting, questioning, and pain. Also, after 14 days of watching his already frail little body waste away, I wish someone had reminded us that Joey's death did not occur from starvation or dehydration, but that the underlying condition, a fatal genetic disorder, ultimately took his life.

Initially fueled by frustration and desperation, my husband and I advocated hard for our youngest son. We questioned the benefit of certain tests and therapies. We demanded more frequent and better communication. When Joey's doctors avoided difficult topics and conversations, we threw the lasso and reeled them back in with raw, honest, and sometimes unsolicited comments. We are grateful for Neil, Joey's neurologist's insight and courage to address a difficult topic at a most difficult time. Without him, Sam and I would have been ill prepared for a traumatic, but normal death. His willingness to work through discomfort and pain made for deep trust and came to serve as the cornerstone in all our communication and interactions. The same holds true for John, Joey's pulmonologist. His humility, compassion, and ability to embrace our pain as well as his own helplessness opened our eyes to the importance of connection. Connection makes the lonely feel seen; it fuels the weary and it is the vehicle that takes you from shock and denial to acceptance and surrender. Connection is more important than your ability to fix someone else's problem or take their pain away.

In the end, it was our trust and connection with John, Neil, and the many other providers, not their knowledge and expertise, that ensured a sacred ending to our son's full and beautiful life.

Parent Commentary

This story speaks to the extraordinary relationships we develop with our child's doctors. When our child is born with a life-limiting condition, there are those doctors who will be with us throughout our child's life. It may be the neurologist who follows the progression of our child's disorder or the pulmonologist who manages our child's ventilator or fragile lungs. It may be the palliative care doctor who becomes part of our team at the time of diagnosis or comes on board when we realize that our child's health is declining as a consequence of his underlying disease. There can be no closer relationship with a doctor than when he or she walks with us through our child's diagnosis, disease progression, decline in health, and, ultimately, our child's death.

When we receive a devastating diagnosis for our child, our first reaction is that we want a doctor to fix it. Before entering the world of life-limiting and rare diseases, we always believed that when your child is sick, you make an appointment with the doctor, the doctor applies their knowledge and experience, writes a script, and your child gets better. This is the world the majority of parents live in. It is shocking for a parent to hear that their child has a disease that cannot be "fixed" and will eventually take their child's life.

There is much that doctors can do for our children over the course of their lives. They resolve acute issues, they manage their extensive and ongoing needs to keep them stable, they ease their pain, and they help us give our child the best quality of life possible. However, what can doctors do when our child's disease progresses to the point where there is nothing more medically that can be done to delay our child's inevitable death?

They can show up.

The two doctors in this story showed up in extraordinary ways. There was nothing more they could do for Joey, but they showed up for his parents. They stepped out of their own comfort zone to come into a dying patient's home. While they came into Joey's home medically empty-handed, what they brought with them instead was great compassion. By showing up, they let Joey's parents know that Joey's life mattered to them. They honored the strong connection Joey's parents felt toward them and validated Joey's parents' trust in them. They helped make getting through the impossible possible. The power of trust and compassion cannot be overstated.

When there is nothing more medically a doctor can do for their patient, there is still so much they can do. Doctors can listen, offer words of comfort, answer questions, and simply be there for the family. While not all doctors can (or are even invited to) show up in person at a patient's home, they can still be there—by making a phone call or by sending or responding to an email. Doctors can continue to walk the walk with their patient's family until the very end.

Physician Commentary

This is an extraordinary journey, relayed with great self-insight and compassion. I would like to comment on three themes. In the first, this mother seems to suddenly come to the realization that her son was suffering. This is heart rending. When physicians try to outline what a child's life will be like with a progressive, neurologic disorder, at least while the child (as a baby) still appears pretty normal, this message is hard to hear. It is difficult to believe that the compassionate physicians described here did not, earlier on, try to prepare this family for what the disease progression would look like. What suffering would look like. But often we are not heard, or, as in other stories in this book, we are told we are not offering enough hope. This is an extraordinarily fine line to walk for physicians. Tell the truth but do not take away hope. In the end, every family is different and sees their child differently. It is truly up to the family to decide the path they take, as long as they are armed with the best evidence possible.

The second issue here appears to be the lack of palliative care support. This field in Pediatrics remains understaffed in many places around the country, but a multi-disciplinary palliative care team could have made the last weeks and days of Joey's life so much less distressing to him and the family. It sounds like this family was just on their own, and this should not be happening in our society today.

Finally, for many physicians, when they have nothing else medically to offer, they may instinctively pull back, at least emotionally. Although we try to avoid these terms today, but to lose a patient means to have failed, at least to some. No matter the disease or lack of treatments, many physicians still take the death of a patient as a personal failure. It is supremely hard to show up in the face of failure. I admire the physicians in this story who did show up at the end, perhaps not even realizing what their presence meant to the family. They showed up because they cared and were likely able to suppress the emotional burden on themselves. Physicians do need to put up some walls to protect themselves, but the truly skilled ones can find an opening in the wall, to drop their armor, and be present when it matters most.

I Did Not Have to Fix It

2

I met Alex when he was 2 days old. He was one of twins who, as many twins do, was born prematurely. Alex's brother died soon after being born. Alex endured many of the complications that come with being born prematurely—he had lung problems, he had vision problems, he had hearing problems, he had feeding problems, and he had liver problems. Alex's brain had been damaged by lack of oxygen and a hemorrhage, and as commonly seen in those circumstances, Alex had epilepsy and cerebral palsy.

Alex spent the first 6 months of his life in the Neonatal Intensive Care Unit. In the beginning, there were days when he was close to dying. "He is a fighter," people used to say, as if being ill, or even dying was only for losers. As time went on, Alex stop needing a machine to help him breathe, he then stopped needing to be fed through his veins, and his liver function became stable, if only his brain had kept up with the progress.

Alex's mother was doggedly determined to give her boy every opportunity to go beyond surviving. She did not *just* take care of him, she was an unyielding, even obstinate, advocate. There was no stone she was going to leave unturned. Her assertive advocacy rubbed some clinicians the wrong way. After going through several neurologists, Alex's mother settled on me. I told her that she had a penchant for tall bearded doctors. She just laughed.

Initially, I saw Alex and his mother about every 3 months. As per protocol, the first series of visits were scheduled for 30 minutes. But soon I learned that 30 minutes was not enough to even get over the greetings. Alex's mother always came with a long list of concerns; only a handful were related to my area of expertise. From rashes, to unexplainable movement. From drooling, to naughty behavior. The kid was 6 months old, what kind of naughty behavior can a child his age have?

Alex's clinic visits went from 30 to 60 to 90 minutes in length. Eventually, I gave up trying to predict how long the encounters were going to be and started scheduling Alex at the end of the day. I would much rather stay at the clinic late than make my other patients wait. And so it went that some visits lasted over 2 hours. What did we discuss? Everything. Alex's health of course, but also stories about Alex's sisters, his

© Springer Nature Switzerland AG 2021   9
A. F. Schrooten, B. P. Markovitz, *Shared Struggles*,
https://doi.org/10.1007/978-3-030-68020-6_2

mother's trials to get Alex services and resources, and even politics (done so against conventional wisdom). Then there were those instances where I did not do anything other than listen. The visits ended when Alex's mother decided it was time to leave.

Alex's mother and my relationship had its ups and downs. There were times when I had to remind her of our agreement—I would always be honest with her, no sugar coating, the unadulterated truth. Alex had a permanent brain injury, and while the injury was not progressive, the consequences were. In some of those instances, Alex's mother would become irritated. She would come back and say, "If Alex could only break out from that crumpled body of his, you would see. No more seizures, no more feeding tubes, no more wheelchairs." Those squabbles would be followed by long periods where I would not see Alex. His mother took him to see clinicians at other institutions, some of which I had recommended. Then, for no evident reason, I would find Alex on my schedule. No explanations were necessary. His mother and I would pick our relationship up exactly where we had left it. Like two old friends.

Alex went from a cute little baby to a budding adolescent. He kept *graduating* from one wheelchair to the next size up. Yet his mother insisted on lifting him from the wheelchair and placing him on the examining table all by herself. Once I tried to help, and backed off lest I have my wrist slapped.

As Alex grew, so did his family. I do not know where his parents found the bravery to have two more children. At each visit, I learned something new about the four girls. Grace, the oldest, started middle school, while Rose, the youngest, was in first grade. Alex's mother shared with me pictures from birthdays and vacations, and I always received a Christmas card.

Alex was a personality. I once saw him on the local evening news paying respect to a fallen law enforcement officer. On the day of his death, the police department of the suburb where Alex lived made him an honorary policeman.

Alex died on an ordinary January day. He fell prey to the flu. One of his sisters brought the virus home from school and soon thereafter, every member of the household was running a fever and sneezing. Alex became acutely ill and was soon admitted to the intensive care unit. But his body was tired. He had been battling all sorts of maladies throughout his life and had finally met his match. Alex's parents wanted the family to send him off in the manner in which he had lived. His mother gave the young man a sponge bath with the assistance of his sisters. Then everyone stood by Alex's bed and had pictures taken. Eventually, Alex's nurse placed him in the arms of his mother and the tube that tethered him to this world was removed.

Starting with medical school and continuing with residency and fellowship, physicians are taught to mend broken bodies. We prescribe medications and do surgery to fulfill our role of healers. To an extent, it is a role with which we are comfortable. Every so often, however, we are asked to take on roles which can make some uncomfortable—listeners, confidants, and consolers. Alex's mother challenged me, and by doing so she made me a better physician. She wanted me to continue performing the responsibilities of healer, as she simultaneously persuaded me to become a member of the family, even if a distant one. What a privilege. A stranger who happened to have been on call the day that Alex was born was invited into a family in pain's ambit.

Alex's wake took place on a miserable winter day. It was cold and snowing. On my way there I called my wife and told her "I will get there, pay my respects, stay for a few minutes and leave. Half-an-hour at most. I'll make it back for our dinner reservations." Boy was I wrong! The line to see Alex snaked through every room of the mortuary—and it was moving slowly. "It will take me an hour tops," I thought "No problem with dinner." Two hours later I called my wife again, "Cancel the dinner plans" I said.

I was finally able to enter the room where Alex was resting. Alex's parents each gave me a hug, and his mother called me "my love." I told them what an honor it had been to be Alex's neurologist. What a privilege it had been to know their family for over 10 years. What a joy it had been to see the girls grow up. As I looked at Alex in his coffin, I recalled the instance when his mother told me "If Alex could only break out from that crumpled body of his." She was right. Alex's body was no longer crumpled. He was resting with composure and dignity.

"Thanks so much for coming to say goodbye to Alex," his mother said. "I can't tell you how much the visits with you meant. I realize I asked you many questions that had nothing to do with neurology, and yet, you always obliged. But most of all, I appreciate that you were willing to listen, to become part of our family, and that you did not feel compelled to try to *fix it*."

Parent Commentary

Admittedly, parents of medically complex children can be obstinate advocates and unlikeable at times. We are often referred to as "that parent." However, it is important to understand that we are unyielding because there are so many people we encounter who put up barriers, treat us as if we are clueless, tell us "no," and make caring for our child extraordinarily difficult. These people are not necessarily the physicians who care for our child. They can be the insurance company, medical equipment company, nursing agency, and school district. If we do not learn to be assertive and stand our ground, our child would not get what they need and are entitled to. It is not personal; it is survival.

The physician who can form a bond with a parent who is fierce, stubborn, and difficult, and who recognizes that every emotion and action is directed toward our child's best interest, is a truly special person. The physician in this story exemplifies this. He is remarkably patient, compassionate, and humble. The bond between a parent and their medically fragile child is inexplicably different than the typical parent-child bond. We are one in the same with our child. Therefore, when our child comes under a physician's care—the physician not only cares for our child, he cares for us. This physician used his medical knowledge and skill to care for Alex; he used his heart to care for Alex's mother. He gave her comfort by listening to her and giving her an extraordinary amount of his time. And he maintained her trust because he was always honest.

Even when we hear what we do not want to hear when it comes to our child's health and prognosis, deep down, we always want honesty from our child's physician. This physician did not take it personally when Alex's mother boycotted him because she did not like what he had to say. As the messenger of news we do not want to hear, physicians often take the brunt of our frustration and despair, even though it is not the messenger we do not like, it is the message. This physician understood that.

Alex's mother knew that there was nothing that any physician could do to "fix" her son. What she needed—what all parents of children with "unfixable" medical conditions need, is a physician who is willing to simply listen to what life with our child entails; how we are impacted; our challenges and our joys. We need to feel supported and understood. We want the physicians caring for our child to know what our life is like outside of the walls of the clinic or hospital and to know us as people, not simply as patients. And when our child dies, there is no greater act of compassion than when our child's physician attends our child's funeral. It means our child's life mattered, and in the end, it all really comes down to that single acknowledgment—our child's life mattered.

Physician Commentary

This is what physicians should aspire to be like. As a pediatric anesthesia and critical care physician, this type of relationship is harder to achieve, as I do not "see" outpatients. But we all see medically complex children regularly, as they often need frequent procedures or ICU admissions. In our financially driven medical system in the United States, for a physician to simply allow whatever time it takes to engage a patient and their family is, alas, all too uncommon. Whether inpatient or outpatient physicians, our "productivity" is being tracked more precisely than ever. Making connections with children and their parents, as this physician did, does not show up on a productivity dashboard. But this is no excuse not to listen, and really hear. Steven Covey, author of *Seven Habits of Highly Successful People* and a visionary in the "leadership" world, succinctly states: First, seek to understand.

I try to regularly practice this mantra: you have two ears and one mouth; you should use them in that proportion. This physician listened, really listened. Parents of these complex children know physicians do not always have answers or solutions, but at least they can listen. It is one of the most basic of human needs: to be heard. It is particularly illustrative that this physician never notes a single intervention or recommendation that was a medical treatment for this child. He recognizes his role as a partner on a journey. A journey that, like all relationships, can have its ups and downs. Yet he stuck it out, literally to the end, and this child's mother recognized that the connection was at least as important, if not more so, than any intervention he recommended.

No Wrong Decisions

3

Morning rounds in the Pediatric Intensive Care Unit (PICU) began at 8 am. Around 7:45 am, parents are told they must leave their critically ill child's bedside and be out of the PICU while rounds take place. This was at a time when PICU beds were separated by thin curtains, and family-centered care was not the standard.

One morning as I waited impatiently in the hallway outside the PICU doors during rounds, I was drawn to a bulletin board displaying pictures of PICU "graduates." I intensely studied each picture and could not help but notice that many of the kids had a small white tube protruding from their necks—a tracheostomy (trach) tube. As I was standing there, my son's cardiothoracic surgeon walked by. I commented that seeing all the kids with trachs did not give me a warm fuzzy feeling. He smiled and said, "I don't think you have anything to worry about."

My 4-month-old son, Jack, was in the PICU for the third time in as many months. His first admission followed an apneic episode at home where he stopped breathing. He was transported to Children's Hospital by ambulance. It was my first experience in an intensive care unit and to say I was shell-shocked is an understatement. The lights were bright, there were multitudes of medical people milling around in a very small space, and alarms were going off all around me. It was overwhelming.

It was discovered during Jack's first PICU admission that he was born with a vascular ring—an anomaly of his aorta. His aorta arched to the right (normal is to the left) forming a ring with a major artery in his upper chest. The vascular ring compressed his trachea and esophagus—which explained his breathing and eating difficulties. Jack had surgery to divide the vascular ring and he was discharged from the hospital 2 weeks after surgery. However, he was only home for 2 days when we had to take him back to the emergency department because he was struggling to breathe. He was readmitted to the PICU. During this admission it was discovered that his right diaphragm was elevated and not moving—likely the result of damage to his phrenic nerve caused during surgery to divide the vascular ring. After 3 more weeks in the hospital, he was discharged home on nasal CPAP and oxygen. Two weeks later, he was admitted to the PICU for the third time because of respiratory distress. This time, Jack was intubated and placed on a ventilator.

© Springer Nature Switzerland AG 2021
A. F. Schrooten, B. P. Markovitz, *Shared Struggles*,
https://doi.org/10.1007/978-3-030-68020-6_3

One week after he was admitted, the first attempt was made to wean Jack off the ventilator and remove his breathing tube. He was unable to successfully breathe on his own and had to be reintubated and put back on the ventilator. After Jack's failed attempt off the ventilator, I heard the word "tracheostomy" mentioned for the first time. My mind immediately went to the bulletin board in the hallway and the pictures of all the kids with trachs. The thought terrified me and I did not want to even consider it.

Jack's elevated diaphragm seemed the most likely explanation for his episodes of respiratory distress. The PICU team suggested surgery to plicate (tack down) the diaphragm, hoping that it would resolve the persistent collapse of Jack's right lung. We willingly agreed to surgery, hoping it would be the fix he needed to get off the ventilator. A few days after surgery, a second attempt was made to remove Jack from the ventilator. He only lasted a few hours before he was in distress and had to be reintubated for the second time. At this point, Jack had been in the PICU and intubated for almost a month, but my husband and I could not bring ourselves to consent to tracheostomy surgery until the doctors could tell us exactly why Jack needed a trach. We needed a diagnosis or some concrete explanation to support what we felt was a drastic intervention.

Given our reluctance to agree to a trach without more information, the PICU team asked for neurology to see Jack. It was observed that he had low tone and muscle weakness, but they did not know if his weakness was due to his prematurity and all the surgeries he had been through in his short life or whether it might be due to an underlying disease. After conducting several bedside strength tests, the neurologist recommended Jack have a muscle biopsy to look for a potential muscle disease.

After agreeing to the muscle biopsy, I was approached by both the PICU intensivist and the attending pulmonologist with their opinions on what they thought we should do. After morning rounds were finished, the intensivist came over to Jack's bed to talk with me. He strongly suggested we consent to the trach and have the surgery done at the same time Jack was under anesthesia for the muscle biopsy. I told him that we needed more information before we could agree to a trach and wanted to wait until the results of the muscle biopsy were known.

He said to me, "If Jack was in an adult ICU you wouldn't have a choice, he would have been trached within the first week and moved out of the ICU."

All I could think to say was, "Well I'm glad Jack is not an adult."

Later that same day, the pulmonologist came to talk with me. He told me he thought it was a good idea to wait for the results of the muscle biopsy. He reasoned that, depending on what we learned, we might not want to intervene at all if Jack had a fatal disease. This was the first time the possibility of Jack not surviving was raised. I was caught off guard by his suggestion. While I strongly pushed for more information, the thought of doing nothing and allowing Jack to die had not entered my mind. The one thing I was sure of, despite our resistance to the trach, was that ultimately we would do what was best for Jack. We wanted him to leave the hospital and come home to his family.

The preliminary results of the muscle biopsy suggested Jack had an inflammatory myopathy, but no specific disease was identified. He was started on a high dose of steroids to see if it would help him regain the strength he needed to successfully wean off the ventilator. After 3 weeks of steroids, another attempt was made to take him off the ventilator. Jack appeared to be doing well breathing on his own for a good part of a day, but by evening, he started showing signs of respiratory distress. Another failed attempt. He was again intubated and put back on the ventilator.

After nearly 3 months in the PICU and multiple failed attempts at getting Jack off the ventilator, I resigned myself to the fact that there was nothing more we could do to stay the trach decision any longer. The only way Jack was ever going to get home was with a trach. Shortly after they reintubated him for the third time, my husband and I agreed to the trach. The PICU staff could not get the consent form prepared fast enough, no doubt fearing that I might change my mind. My hand shook as I signed the consent; I was disheartened and scared.

After Jack came out of surgery, I stood at his bedside just trying to take it all in. He was sleeping peacefully, his beautiful face free from tape and tubes for the first time in over 3 months, having now been replaced by a white tube protruding from his neck. As I was standing there, one of the critical care fellows came over and stood next to me. I did not have any recollection of meeting her before, but she must have been part of Jack's care team. Certain of what she was thinking, I said to her, "I guess you're glad we finally agreed to the trach." Her response was not what I was expecting to hear. She said, "You haven't made one wrong decision regarding Jack." At that moment, I felt a tremendous weight lift off my shoulders. Any reservations and guilt that I had about taking so long to make the decision to trach Jack were immediately extinguished by her kind and supportive words.

Those months Jack spent in the PICU were some of the most difficult months of my life. Every 2 weeks the team of doctors changed and with each turnover came differing views and differing approaches. We were there so long that eventually the teams circled back. I am certain there were some who were growing impatient with us. I felt pressured by some teams to make a decision while other teams supported our need to explore every possible option before consenting to the trach surgery.

I recognize time is a precious commodity in an intensive care environment, both in terms of cost and the need to free up the bed for other critical patients. If we had consented at the first mention of a trach, Jack's stay would have been shortened by at least 2 months. However, despite what the intensive care team may have thought, it was not a simple decision. It was a decision that would have a significant impact on Jack's life and our family's life. My husband and I both worked full time, we had two other children at home, and we lived thousands of miles away from extended family. How were we going to care for a child with a trach (and ventilator), care for our two other children, and keep our jobs? Who was going to help us? It was not as simple as "give my child a trach and then we'll go home." The consequences of the decision were overwhelming and profoundly life altering for our entire family.

In retrospect, it feels selfish to have taken up valuable ICU space and resources for so many months, especially given that the trach was ultimately the right decision and an important part of why Jack survived and thrived for the 15 years he was with us. However, at the time, I only knew that I needed some certainty before I could make any decisions—an unrealistic expectation, in hindsight.

I will always be grateful for the words shared by the PICU fellow who joined me at Jack's bedside after his trach surgery. She understood how difficult a decision it was for us to agree to the trach and she showed great compassion by validating our decision-making process rather than judging us. Her compassion in that moment is something I have never forgotten. While I never saw that doctor again, 20 years later, I still remember her name.

Parent Commentary

When asking parents to make a decision of whether to pursue a surgery or intervention for their seriously ill child, I believe it is important to take into consideration these questions: how much is known and unknown about the child's condition and prognosis, about the family, and about the short-term and long-term consequences of the decision? The answers to these questions can provide some insight to how complicated the decision is for the parents.

In the case of whether to consent to a tracheostomy for our child, the parent is agreeing to so much more than a relatively simple surgery. Jack's parents were asked to make a decision that would have long-term and significant implications for not only Jack's quality of life, but his entire family's quality of life. And this decision had to be made without having a diagnosis or prognosis for their son. Physicians have seen enough to know that there is much uncertainty in medicine and decisions often have to be made in the face of the unknown. Nevertheless, it is human nature to want certainty and predictability when making decisions, even more so when it comes to decisions involving our child's health and life. Parents need to feel supported throughout the decision-making process. Not only are parents having to make difficult and life-altering decisions, they have to make those decisions while they are simultaneously grieving the loss of a healthy child and the life they expected and wanted. The weight of this emotional burden is indescribable.

When parents are asked to make a decision that will significantly impact their child's life and their family's life long after they leave the confines of the hospital, and when those decisions have to be made in the face of the unknown, parents should be given the time they need, and they should never be made to feel pressured to make their decision. Decisions that may seem routine and straightforward to a physician can be herculean to the parents who have to make them. Please be patient with us.

Physician Commentary

Uncertainty is the bane of our existence as physicians. The world paints us as human; we can make mistakes and be wrong, but uncertainty about a diagnosis and therefore the prognosis is not something most people think of when they think about doctors. Certainly, many diagnoses are indeed certain and if the diagnosis is common enough, painting at least a reasonable range of possible outcomes is manageable. But many of the children discussed in this book either have rare diseases or complex conditions where predicting outcomes is educated guesswork at best. We are on the precipice of personalized medicine, where we can much more reliably pin down a diagnosis to the specific genetic mutation. However, knowing exactly what genetic code piece is broken, if it is a rare condition, may not really help predict a child's outcome. Even relying on a textbook is fraught with uncertainty, since we do not know what it means when they say: children with x disease usually die before their first birthday. How many children? What interventions were undertaken for them? Did they die despite "everything" being done, or were the prophesies self-fulfilling by allowing the "inevitable" to occur. It is a vexing problem.

In this child's case, there really was not a satisfactory diagnosis. Every effort was made to "wean" the baby from the ventilator, and some correctable conditions were addressed, but the baby was still stuck. From a medical standpoint (in Pediatrics), there is no right answer as to when to acknowledge that staying in the PICU with an endotracheal tube is simply not acceptable any longer. A tracheostomy allows mobility, security of the airway, and even possibly the ability to eat by mouth. But as was pointed out, the impact of the decision to perform a tracheostomy and use a portable ventilator has a profound impact on the entire family. This decision should never be rushed and should be done in a multidisciplinary fashion, including the physician team (usually pulmonary specialists) that will be directing the care of the child after he or she leaves the PICU. Only they have the insight into how to counsel families on what it might be like to have a child at home on a ventilator.

It comes back to diagnoses and prognoses. With many children, they can literally grow out of the condition that causes their chronic respiratory failure. Others have known progressive diseases, where the expectation to wean from mechanical support is less likely. But if we do not even know what the diagnosis is, how can we advise on a course of action. And if uncertainty over a diagnosis haunts physicians, imagine how our families feel. This story tells us just that.

Reuniting Families

4

I am part of a pediatric pulmonary division that includes a large and long-standing program designed to send children with chronic respiratory failure home on ventilators. I like to say that the unofficial motto of the program is "we reunite families." I arrived at this realization over time and via my experiences working with children who are in such tenuous respiratory conditions that without life support they would die, and without a program to provide this in the community, they would never be able to leave the hospital. In the beginning of my career, my focus was much more on the nuts and bolts of figuring out the best settings on the ventilator and making sure we could do this therapy safely. However, with time, I developed a deeper understanding of the importance of being at home for our patients and the need for mothers and fathers and brothers and sisters to be together under one roof, even if only for a short time. One family in particular brought this realization home to me.

Children born with spina bifida, a birth defect of the spine and spinal cord, occasionally have such severe injury to their brain that they develop respiratory failure. The brain cannot send the information to nerves to activate the breathing muscles. This type of brain injury means that other features of brain control that we tend to take for granted, like increases in heart rate and blood pressure in response to stress, are also out of commission. In this circumstance, even when we support breathing with a ventilator, there is a very high risk of babies dying from something else—like otherwise treatable infections. In fact, the first dozen babies with this extreme form of spina bifida that we treated for respiratory failure all passed away despite being on a ventilator.

When I met little Rachel and her mother, Maria, it seemed pretty straightforward to me what I would recommend. Rachel was a baby with spina bifida who could not breathe on her own. She had a tube in her throat connected to a ventilator. Placing a tracheostomy (a surgically placed airway in the windpipe) only to watch her die with her first respiratory tract infection did not seem like a good plan. Withdrawing the ventilator and keeping her comfortable seemed the better course of action.

© Springer Nature Switzerland AG 2021
A. F. Schrooten, B. P. Markovitz, *Shared Struggles*,
https://doi.org/10.1007/978-3-030-68020-6_4

I met with Maria and the rest of the team, and I shared with her our experience with other babies like Rachel. Maria wanted time to think about her decision and we agreed to meet again. It was hard on the team to only have such grim and limited options to offer, but of course unimaginably hard for the family.

When we met again at the bedside, Maria asked me if we would not be willing to try the option for the tracheostomy and the ventilator. She understood that there would be a risk that Rachel might not do well with the surgery and that even if we were able to send her home it would likely be only for a little while. Maria must have seen the concern and perhaps resistance on my face, and she took my hand and said, "Doctora, my children, they stand by the empty crib and they cry." This image was so poignant. I took the lead in convincing the rest of the health care team that going home to her family was the pathway we would take for Rachel.

Rachel was able to have her tracheostomy placed and her mother and father learned all of the needed care. This is no small undertaking because we ask parents to assume the tasks that registered nurses and respiratory care practitioners perform in the hospital. Rachel was able to go home to her family, sleep in her crib, and be with her brother and sister.

I wish that this was a story with a miracle ending, and in a way it is, but I cannot tell you that Rachel beat the odds and had a long life with her family. She spent about 6 months at home, however, with her first infection she developed shock and acute respiratory failure.

She was in our Pediatric ICU, and the intensive care team felt that there was no chance for her to survive this illness. She was on medications to support her blood pressure and her heart and lungs were failing. Maria understood the situation. She knew it was time for Rachel to leave this world for the next. She had expressed a desire to donate any of Rachel's organs that might help another child. Maria only had one small request. She asked that we delay the removal of life support until Rachel's grandmother could get to the ICU to meet her granddaughter for the first time. She was on her way and would be there the next morning. I sat with Maria and held Rachel's hand. I promised I would talk to the ICU team about the timing for removing life support.

I went to find the on-call doctor, but the ICU was very busy that night, there seemed to be emergencies in every room and I did not want to interrupt. I went back to Rachel's bedside, but before I could say anything Maria looked at me and said, "Doctora, I see how busy it is here and how all the beds are full. I don't want to take a bed away from a child that needs it, whose life can be saved. We will say good-bye to Rachel tonight."

That was over 20 years ago, and I have worked with hundreds of children and families since then and have successfully discharged many infants and children in respiratory failure on assisted ventilation home to be with their families. I have supported many families as best I can through difficult and painful decisions when there are no good options for their child. Just like with Rachel and her mother, from each family, I learn a little more and I hope that I become a better doctor with each encounter. I can only feel humbled in the face of the love that parents have not only for their own child, but even for the children of parents they will never meet.

The memory of Rachel's mother and her grace and beauty in the most tragic circumstances is what I hold fast to and try to honor when I say, "we reunite families."

Parent Commentary

As a new parent of a child born with a devastating and life-limiting condition, we are overwhelmed with all the information coming at us regarding our child's diagnosis and prognosis. We are still processing our grief while having to make life-altering decisions for our child. Because we are overwhelmed and do not yet have the experience or knowledge to fully understand the ramifications of our child's diagnosis, we are highly influenced by the medical professionals caring for our child. Parents and physicians both want to do what is in the child's best interest, but the physician and parent may have very different views based on their own belief systems, values, and experiences. The physician has the advantage of experience to know what the child's course will look like both with and without medical intervention. The parents only know that they cannot fathom a life without their child.

Going into the meeting with Rachel's mother, the physician strongly believed that withdrawing support and providing comfort measures was the best course of treatment for Rachel. When Rachel's mother asked for time to think about what she wanted to do, the physician not only honored her wish for more time, she stepped up and became her advocate. When Rachel's mother asked for aggressive medical intervention to allow her daughter to go home and be with her family, the physician pushed to make it happen, despite the fact that it was not the approach she recommended and knowing she would get push back from the team. When Rachel ended up back in the Pediatric ICU and end-of-life decisions had to be made, the physician again supported the parent's wish for more time and was prepared to advocate on her behalf with the team.

In the medical environment, parents need advocates. Parents rely on physicians to provide them with information, options, and recommendations. When a parent makes a decision that is not consistent with the recommendations of the physician or health care team, they can feel unsupported and alone. This physician did not take it personally when Rachel's mother wanted to take a different course than the one she recommended. She gave Rachel's mother an incredible gift by giving her time, respecting her decision, and, most exceptionally, by being her advocate and leading the way to make sure that Rachel was able to go home and spend time surrounded by the love of her family. She helped give Rachel the best life possible during her short time here in earth.

Physician Commentary

There are four pillars of western medical ethics: autonomy (patients get to choose what happens to them), beneficence (the obligation to "do good"), non-maleficence (do not harm the patient), and justice (to treat everyone equitably). Of these, autonomy is the one most unique to modern medicine in our country. In the past, and still in many countries, doctors just decide what is "right" for the patients and patients have little say in the matter. In Pediatrics, we often call this "surrogate autonomy," because parents are given the choice for their children. Unfortunately, to some physicians, in offering choices to patients (good!), they have abrogated their expertise and experience by failing to actually recommend a course of action (not good!). Physicians are still expected to guide patients and families and make a medical recommendation. Particularly in the matter of life and death, a physician should not say something like, "we can do this treatment or no treatment, it is up to you." The physician, using their knowledge and incorporating the patient's and family values, should make a plan they feel is in the patient's best interest. That is what this physician did in recommending that Rachel not receive a tracheostomy and be sent home on a ventilator.

However, given reasonable options, physicians must be flexible and be open to a family choosing the alternate course, as happened in this situation. Once this physician realized what was of paramount importance to the mother, she accepted her decision and supported her and the baby completely.

What strikes me profoundly about this story though was the mother's comment that final evening in the PICU. Thinking selflessly about her and her daughter, she instinctively wanted to help other children by making sure there was room for them to come if needed. Recently I sat with a family whose daughter suffered a drowning event and had severe brain damage from the prolonged cardiac arrest. After informing them of the child's grim prognosis, at that first meeting the grandmother asked if her other organs were okay and could they be donated to another child. Such acts of wanting to help others in moments of profound grief never fail to take my breath away.

Leading with Compassion

5

I went into labor at 30 weeks with my first pregnancy. The same night I was admitted to the hospital, a neonatologist came to talk with me about what to expect if labor could not be stopped and I delivered. He put me at ease, telling me that though it was not ideal and there were a lot of challenges, they rarely lost 30-weekers.

Fortunately, my labor was stopped. After weeks of bed rest and medications, my water broke at 37 weeks. My husband, Jason, and I were so relieved to have made it to full term. We were ready to meet our son or daughter. At the hospital, I was being transferred from the women's evaluation unit to labor and delivery when the same neonatologist happened to step into the elevator with me. I gleefully told him that I had made it and would not need him after all. I thanked him for his calming manner 7 weeks earlier.

Ben's birth and first 24 hours were uneventful. I was concerned breastfeeding was not going well, and Ben seemed very still and quiet most of the time. The nurses reassured me that he was just a sleepy baby and that his Apgars had been great. Friends had come by to visit and I was in bed holding Ben in my arms when I suddenly realized he was turning blue. Ben had stopped breathing. Jason pushed the call button and our friend ran out of the room to scream for help. Before I could react, Ben was whisked out of my arms by a nurse and rushed down the hall to the Neonatal Intensive Care Unit (NICU). Jason ran after them. He saw a crowd of medical personnel gathered around Ben performing CPR. A nurse was standing to the side, shaking her head, and saying, "He's gone. He's gone." Someone noticed Jason standing there and walked him back to my bedside.

Eventually, the neonatologist came to speak with us. He pulled up a chair and sat close, giving us full eye contact. We fully believed he was there to give us the official pronouncement of Ben's death. Instead, he slowly and carefully, with great compassion, gave us the details of Ben's critical status. He told us Ben suffered a cardiac arrest, but he was breathing again with the help of a machine and he had a heartbeat. We put our hands out to stop him in disbelief and asked if we could have a minute to pray. He respectfully and patiently gave us the time we requested. Afterward, he prepared us by explaining how Ben would look and what to expect

© Springer Nature Switzerland AG 2021
A. F. Schrooten, B. P. Markovitz, *Shared Struggles*,
https://doi.org/10.1007/978-3-030-68020-6_5

once we would be allowed to see him. As he left, he hugged us and let us know someone would come back to get us when it was time to see Ben.

Five days after that event, Jason stayed at Ben's NICU bedside while I had lunch with my mom in the hospital cafeteria. We felt confident about Ben's progress and started to relax. I was sitting with my mom in the cafeteria when the hospital chaplain came over and told me Jason needed me to come upstairs because Ben had pulled out his breathing tube. I was not sure how to take this information because I knew the doctors had discussed removing the tube to see how Ben would handle it. Sending a chaplain to fetch me felt ominous.

I got upstairs and saw Jason standing in the hall near the door to the NICU. He was visibly shaken with arms crossed talking with our neonatologist. I knew the news was horrible. Ben had reached up above his head and suddenly pulled down his arm causing his breathing tube to dislodge. He immediately went into another cardiac arrest and no one could do anything about it. The neonatologist told us they had been working on Ben for over 20 minutes, but he was not responding to any of their efforts. He said he needed to get back to Ben to see if there was anything more that could be done. He closed the door and the chaplain directed us to a private conference room. As we walked away, the neonatologist suddenly stuck his head out into the hall again and shouted, "We have a heart beat!" We motioned for him to go back to our son, saying, "Go! Go!"

Later, the neonatologist came to the conference room to explain what had happened. He was visibly emotional. He told us he was very perplexed because what happened with Ben should not have happened. He said babies pull their breathing tubes out all the time and they just put them back in. Usually, everything is fine. In addition, Ben had been doing so well before the second cardiac arrest that the NICU team planned to remove him from the ventilator later that night. Once again, he hugged us as he left the room. I appreciated his frankness and his willingness to acknowledge that he did not know what was happening with Ben. Even more, I appreciated that it was obvious he really cared.

In the following days, Ben continued to have sudden and unexplained significant drops in his oxygen saturations. He no longer breathed over the ventilator. The neonatologist ordered an MRI and warned us he expected bad news. I asked him how we would know if we were being cruel to let Ben continue to struggle. He reassured me by saying, "We are not there yet." His words were so comforting because they let me know this was not about providing heroic medical care just because we could, it was about keeping hope alive. I do not recall the exact details of the MRI, but I recall the sheer joy and surprise in the neonatologist's face when he told us the MRI was unimpressive considering the trauma to Ben's brain from the cardiac arrests, seizures, and frequent drops in oxygen saturations. We were on an emotional roller coaster and the neonatologist seemed to be in the car directly ahead of us, leading the way.

The cause of Ben's sudden drops in oxygen saturations was assumed, but not confirmed, to be some type of airway obstruction. When he was 4 weeks old, Ben had surgery for a tracheostomy. Although he continued to have unexplained desaturations, he could be more easily rescued with the trach. Two weeks after surgery,

Ben was discharged from the NICU and our family of three was under the same roof for the first time since Ben was born.

The neonatologist who cared for Ben during this critical time ushered two very scared parents through the most traumatic experience of their lives with patience, humility, compassion, and probably most notably, a willingness to display his own vulnerability and emotions. Thirteen years later, I reached out to this retired neonatologist with a letter, telling him how much his compassion meant to us in those early days. I wrote:

> I recall many encounters with you that were terrifying because of what Ben was experiencing. But the fact that it was obvious you cared on a level deeper than a mere scientist trying to fix broken parts, I can look back at those moments and still feel the compassion and concern you shared with us. I recall your determined face, your compassionate words, your kind touch, your tearful eyes and your joyfulness when things went miraculously well. I am moved to share our admiration and gratitude, even if it is a little belated. I want you to know that those moments really mattered to us and ministered to us then and still.

He wrote back, touched by the gesture. He had not forgotten that miraculous full termer who beat the odds.

Parent Commentary

Being thrust into a critical care environment with a sick child is a traumatic experience for any parent. The noise, the lights, the barrage of people, the pace—it is all overwhelming. As new parents, we may have spent months leading up to our child's birth researching and interviewing different physicians to find the best pediatrician for our child. Then suddenly, our child's life is in the hands of a physician we have never met before and who we know nothing about. There is little opportunity to establish a relationship with the physician before technical, unfamiliar, and scary information concerning our child is conveyed. How a physician communicates in this limited window of opportunity is instrumental in gaining the parent's trust and can make all the difference in how information is received, processed, and accepted. Choice of words, tone, and body language all matter.

The neonatologist in this story stands out for many reasons. He sat down with Ben's parents; he gave them eye contact and his full attention. By his attentiveness and compassion, he created a space that gave these parents time to absorb the information and ask questions at a pace that allowed them to understand what was going on with their son. This set the foundation for a trusting relationship. When Ben's condition was uncertain, his mother trusted this physician enough to ask the tough question of whether they were doing the right thing by continuing treatment and, more significantly, she trusted his answer that it was not yet time to make difficult decisions.

This physician openly displayed his emotions. We all know that doctors are human too, but it is a side that is not often revealed. When our child is critically ill in an intensive care environment and things are happening fast all around us, we are scared and vulnerable. Yes, we want a physician who has the technical excellence to help our child, but we also want a physician who is caring. Thirteen years later, it is his compassion, his touch, his tears, and his joy—his human qualities—that this physician is most remembered and cherished for.

Physician Commentary

This family's story about their newborn son who suffered several cardiac arrests sends a powerful message to me as a pediatric intensivist—a pediatrician who works in the Pediatric ICU. Although this baby was a newborn and cared for in a Neonatal ICU by a neonatologist, this does not dilute the impact of the message. This story conveys how powerfully profound a human connection between a physician and parents of ill children can be and how quickly this connection can be made. The simple act of sitting down at eye level with parents is critical to this bonding. This physician also showed emotion. He conveyed that he genuinely cared about the patient and his parents. He took his time with explanations. By allowing the moment the parents requested to pray, he showed true respect for Ben's parents as individuals, not just recipients of information.

The analogy they used about being on an emotional roller coaster with the physician riding along right in front of them struck me in way that I have never heard before, but I instantly related to this with some serious "been there" moments coming to mind.

Not once do the parents mention this physician's technical expertise, training, or medical knowledge. The bond they formed with him and the trust they put in him was because of his attitude and behavior, not because of his actual technical expertise. Obviously, he must have been a qualified physician, but what "qualified" him in their hearts and minds was how much he cared and how he related to them as a compassionate person. It calls to mind the adage we talk about—though not enough—in medicine: "Patients do not care about how much you know until they know how much you care."

Minute by Minute, Step by Step

6

It was unusual to be called to the operating room for a code blue. I ran, just as I do every time my pager beeps. This time was different because it was off-unit in a foreign environment with unfamiliar team members. The race continued when my charge nurse, attending, and I arrived at the operating room doors. Who could put on the white bunny suit, mask, and blue cap fastest? As we rushed into the sterile environment, the operating room team was giving our teenage patient another dose of epinephrine. Yelling over the large crowd, the anesthesiologist presented the patient to us. On their turf, my calm and collected ICU attending introduced herself and explained she would be leading the code now.

I stood next to her, taking in everything. I watched the rate of compressions, humming the Bee Gee's "Staying Alive" to make sure our line of chest compressors stayed on beat. More people entered, watching silently. The operating room documenter shouted out the time since last medication and pulse check. The operating room pharmacists continued to draw up medications: epinephrine, calcium, sodium bicarbonate. For a moment, I watched the clock and noticed the red second hand moving slower for a beat, and then skip 2. Our patient progressively became more bruised on her chest.

After 45 minutes, the documenter came to our side to let us know how much time had passed, knowing his simple statement hinted at a loaded question. Until what time would we be continuing chest compressions? The time spoke for itself.

With a pit in my stomach, I asked my attending, "Has anyone updated the family?"

My attending motioned for the surgeon to come close to her so they could have a semi-private conversation amidst the masses. My attending explained that it was almost time to call time of death—the formal transition between life and death. The surgeon responded that he was not yet ready.

Ready to stop compressions?

Ready to face reality?

I had so many questions, but all I said was, "You don't have to update the family alone. I'll go with you."

© Springer Nature Switzerland AG 2021
A. F. Schrooten, B. P. Markovitz, *Shared Struggles*,
https://doi.org/10.1007/978-3-030-68020-6_6

Together we walked to the waiting room to meet the only parents left at this hour. Their faces lit up as the surgeon approached. His was a friendly face they had known throughout years of surgeries for their daughter's fragile bones from a longstanding muscle disease.

He quietly sat down and explained, "We lost her, and I don't know why."

The parents howled. Dad paced the room; mom sat shocked.

"But it was an elective procedure. What happened?"

The surgeon explained technicalities. "We were closing her wound and then we lost her blood pressure."

I explained that the operating room was full of people trying to bring their daughter back to life, but at this point there was nothing more we could do. I invited our patient's parents into the operating room so that they could be with their daughter and part of the team. Shuffling from the waiting room to the operating room across the shiny linoleum floor felt like an eternity. Arm in arm, I carried mom's weight alongside my body and on my mind. Like a broken record, I reiterated there was nothing our patient's mother did wrong or could have done differently. It was not her fault. She asked me how she could keep going. Out loud, I said, "Minute by minute, step by step." Internally, I gave myself the same talk.

As we entered the operating room, I recognized four faces—three nurses from the PICU and my attending. The rest of the room, nearly forty people now, were strangers that formed our team. It was this team that worked together to perfuse our patient's body. Between the blue hat and white mask, it was the eyes of these individuals who watched our patient's parents embrace their child for the last time. The room was silent, except for dad's cries.

Like a great Greek tragedy in the center of this amphitheater, we watched the scene unfold. My attending said, "I'm so sorry. There's nothing more we can offer. We have tried everything." And with that, compressions stopped.

With the surgeon, I walked our patient's parents up to the ICU to allow for a more intimate goodbye. We gave our patient's mother and father privacy as they cleansed their daughter's body. I came to learn this was a nightly ritual in their home for the last decade. However, this night would be their last. They massaged their daughter's beautiful dark hair, washed blood away from fresh wounds, and were thoughtful in the way they moved from one contractured limb to the next.

Our team took these moments to introduce ourselves and debrief. I learned that in over 30 years of practice, our surgeon had never had to tell a family their child died. The level of compassion that swelled the room impressed me. Each of us thanked our unfamiliar partners, sharing moments that will never be forgotten. We ended the debrief with a moment of silence to honor our patient.

This was the beginning of my shift that night. The details of the operating room stayed with me every moment of those 14 hours. The chaplain asked me how I was doing. I bit my lower lip, nodded. I asked her to ask me again tomorrow. The rest of the night was a blur.

The next day I called my family and told them I love them. I tried to explain the events from the preceding night, but they did not quite understand. I felt isolated. I wrote as a way to cope, slept a few hours, and walked out the door.

The afternoon was raw and cold. The hospital loomed in the distance. A sudden gust of wind rose up from the lake and slowed my heavy footsteps. Suddenly I did not know how I could possibly keep going. I heard the guttural sobs from the waiting room, saw the sad shining eyes above the surgical masks, the parents holding each other in a twisted knot of pain and love. Then, I listened to my voice, in the hallway, in my head: "Minute by minute. Step by step."

The light turned green. I continued on.

As I reflect on the experience, I regret one moment. After the debrief with the operating room personnel, my co-fellow offered to hold my pager for 15 minutes so I could have a short reprieve from being called to help with another patient. I said, "No." Would providing an ounce of compassion for myself have been a sign of weakness? Was continuing on, as if nothing happened, a sign of strength? Compassion exuded from my soul for this family, almost to the point that I could no longer continue on. But for myself, it was held captive, deep in the pit within my stomach. I *needed* a moment to remind myself I am human too. However, in the moment, it was not something I *wanted* to admit. For the future, it is something I will embrace.

Parent Commentary

Compassion is talked about a lot in the delivery of health care. We want the doctors caring for our children to show compassion to our child and to us. When doctors show compassion, we remember it. When doctors fail to show compassion, we remember it. Because our child is the one suffering and because we suffer when our child suffers, we only see compassion within the narrow confines of our individual world of suffering and how it impacts us and our child.

This story is an important and impactful reminder that compassion in health care extends well beyond the patient and family. This doctor extended compassion to the family when she asked in the operating room if the family had been updated. She extended compassion as she walked arm in arm with the patient's mother back to the operating room. But beyond that, she also extended compassion to the surgeon when she told him he did not have to update the family alone and when she accompanied him to the waiting room. The operating team extended compassion to each other during their debriefing time, as they introduced themselves and thanked each other. This doctor displayed extraordinary compassion to everyone involved in this tragic event. Yet, at the end of a difficult shift, she failed to extend compassion to herself.

It is important for parents and patients to recognize that we are only one of many challenging encounters and experiences a doctor has in any given day. We have seen the sad and horrific outcomes for families that unfold in emergency rooms, intensive care units, and surgery waiting rooms, hoping that we never have to go through what we are witnessing. Doctors have to experience these outcomes day in and day out with their patients and families. We expect and deserve to be treated with compassion by our child's doctors. We should also extend compassion in return because, even if they do not expect it, doctors deserve to be treated with compassion too.

Physician Commentary

The emotional toll that physicians bear as they deal with intense, life and death situations has never been fully addressed. We are humans too, and we feel the pain when there is a loss in front of us. There is a great deal of attention now to physician well-being and burnout, but the sources of these issues are not, in large part, due to our patient outcomes. They relate more to loss of physician autonomy, administrative burdens, long hours, etc. When we lose a patient, we feel the searing pain, but we tell ourselves (subconsciously usually) that our pain is nothing compared to what the family is experiencing. So, we engage in the game of comparative pain, which is highly counterproductive. Pain is not a zero-sum game; there is plenty to go around. Fortunately, so is compassion. Because we demonstrate empathy and compassion for our patients and families does not mean there is no compassion left for ourselves. There is no one-size-fits-all solution for self-compassion. In my anecdotal experience, a good cry is a good start.

Seek Permission First

7

We needed to find a new craniofacial team for our 8-year-old daughter, Emma. My job transferred us across the country, and the logistics of staying connected with the team in New York was going to be prohibitive in terms of both time and costs. Emma was born with Arnold's syndrome—a craniofacial disorder that manifests in abnormal bone development and often requires multiple surgeries to correct. At eight, Emma's medical journey had already been long and difficult, and she knew more about absorbing pain and pushing through countless medical procedures than most people learn in their entire lives. Emma was astonishingly resilient and had a toughness any linebacker could only aspire to; however, even from her earliest years she was also incredibly gentle, especially toward children and she showed true empathy toward another child hurt or in distress.

My wife, Annie, scheduled an initial meeting with the multidisciplinary craniofacial team at a premier teaching hospital for children that was closer to where we were now living. We stayed overnight in a nearby hotel and arrived early the next morning to begin the registration, insurance, and documentation tasks before we met the first of many disciplines throughout the day. Emma was well used to examinations, both physical and psychological, but having her 6-year-old sister Enya with her made the numerous appointments and wait times so much easier to bear.

The final appointment of the day was at 3:30 in the afternoon with the plastic surgeon—the lead for the craniofacial team. We expected that the doctor would meet Emma, make the obligatory examination, and later meet with me and Annie to discuss Emma's care plan. Things do not always turn out as expected. We waited in a small examination room, Emma sat on the bed, and Annie sat in the chair beside her. I looked out the window over downtown and was caught by the brightness of the sun, and, from the vantage point of the twelfth floor of the hospital, I could see a distinct layer of haze over the downtown area. As a runner, I wondered what the effects of breathing that air must be like when running.

When the door finally opened, the surgeon entered the room with six or seven residents in tow. He introduced himself to us and spoke kindly to Emma, who sat impatiently, wanting to be done with all of this so she could join her sister, who was

© Springer Nature Switzerland AG 2021   31
A. F. Schrooten, B. P. Markovitz, *Shared Struggles*,
https://doi.org/10.1007/978-3-030-68020-6_7

playing and making friends in the playroom down the corridor. Suddenly, the conversation became a teaching moment as the surgeon began pointing at Emma's facial features and describing them as abnormal, but typical of her syndrome. Her jaw, the cranium, eyes, ears all appeared to be a target. For a moment, that seemed to last forever, I stood behind the group of residents in total shock at the words being used in front of my young daughter—a girl of high intelligence who was learning much too quickly how different she was. I saw Annie looking stunned and saw big tears welling up in Emma's eyes.

Loudly and clearly I exclaimed, "There's a lot of pollution here, isn't there?" Every head turned back to look at me and wonder at the interruption of the surgeon's detailed description of the subject. I maneuvered my way through the residents to the bed, picked Emma up, kissed her on the cheek, and gave her a little pat as I let her out the door and told her to find her sister and go play.

I have been accused of "flat-lining" in times of crisis; however, this was not one of them. I was visibly upset as I asked the surgeon if he realized that the medical terms and description he used fell like thunder on an impressionable and innocent young mind. The residents were soon dismissed and the surgeon attempted to rationalize the barrage he had just conducted. Annie diplomatically stepped in and suggested that it had been a long day and that we could wait for the team's report and care plan as we needed to get going to feed the girls dinner.

Once in the car, Annie's emotions unraveled. To keep the atmosphere in the back seat exciting and happy, I put on the girls' favorite Raffi CD, but Annie was getting ever more upset at the surgical team's treatment of Emma in the most impersonal way imaginable.

Emma was at the age of awareness and self-discovery and we knew one day she would be hit with a reality she would not be prepared for. Annie and I had talked about this many times both in private and with the counselors on Emma's care team. Emma is an intelligent well-adjusted child and our goal was never to hide her from the world or the world from her, but to arm her with knowledge and understanding as she grew and was able to comprehend how her medical condition made her special. Our family is blessed in love and Annie's and my focus was always centered on the family. With respect to Emma's medical condition, we took the attitude that there was a whole lot more right with her than there was wrong. We hoped and prayed we were providing a love-filled, positive acceptance of others without fault or prejudice. There were always those incidences that Annie and I were on guard for, the stares, the unthinking remarks, and sometimes the cruel ones, and we usually did a good job shielding Emma from the worst of what could be thrown at her in the public space. That is why we were caught so off-guard in the surgeon's office by the overly critical inspection and words used to describe the physical with no regard to the psychological impact on our beautiful little girl. Now in the car, in the wake of what had just occurred, Annie and I both felt we had somehow failed and had let Emma down. We failed to anticipate and intercede like we were primed to do in public. We understood the surgeon and medical staff meant neither harm nor disrespect, but even as we replayed it, we were shocked at the lack of empathy and human kindness in substitution for high-minded, fact-based analysis.

Later, at the restaurant where we were having dinner, the waitress generously let the girls run untethered through the closed off section of the restaurant while Annie and I talked. We tried to put into perspective how better to protect our daughter from unthinking and insensitive words, especially from the most unexpected source—her own medical care team. Throughout this amazingly wonderful journey our family has been on because of our daughter, we have visited many hospitals across the United States looking for the specialists that could best treat the myriad of ailments that often go along with Emma's syndrome. It is curious, while each medical center has health care as a core value and patient well-being as a tenet, there is a distinct culture and a different "personality" or feeling in each place. Some centers appear to be exceptionally well trained in the psychosocial aspect of the child-doctor-family triad and well versed in the numerous and delicate factors that go into communicating with the child. The child's age, intelligence, acceptance, maturity, and understanding are all subjective but critical aspects that must be weighed by the medical team in the first precious moments of introduction and meeting the child-family part of the triad. Just as there is an examination of the patient by the medical care team, there too is an evaluation of all the subjective, yet no less impactful, aspects of the medical team by the family. It takes a well-balanced family-doctor approach to provide the comprehensive medical care, needs, love, and attention that any child deserves to have. This approach is just heightened for children with special health care needs.

Parent Commentary

There are many advantages to receiving care at a teaching hospital. These hospitals are at the forefront of medical education and innovative research. It is where we will find the highly trained and expert physicians and surgeons we want for our child, especially if our child has a rare diagnosis or condition. Depending on where we live, a teaching hospital may be the only choice we have for our child's care. Most parents know that when we bring our child to a teaching hospital, part of the deal is that we have to endure the training component that is an integral part of the care provided. However, the child's best interest should always come before the need to teach. In this teaching encounter, there appeared to be little consideration or sensitivity for a patient who was very much aware of what was being said about her atypical appearance in a room full of strangers.

The better and more compassionate approach would have been to step outside the room to talk with Emma's parents first to find out Emma's level of understanding, to ask if they had any concerns or questions, and to ask permission to conduct the detailed and descriptive exam intended. After talking with the parents, then introduce yourself and take some time to establish rapport with the child. Explain who all the people in the room are and why they are there. Explain what your exam will involve in words the child can understand. Ask the child if she has any questions and ask her permission to begin the exam. When conducting the exam, take your cues from the child and look for signs of anxiety or fear. This surgeon overstepped Emma's threshold for touching, looking, and sharing of information about her appearance. Her tears should have been enough to have stopped the exam. At that point, discussions with the team could have easily taken place outside of the room.

While I am sure that the surgeon never intended to upset Emma, it is somewhat surprising that a doctor who cares for children with craniofacial disorders would not be more sensitive to what he is saying about the child's appearance. The reactions of Emma and her father hopefully raised some awareness on the part of the surgeon about how he approaches teaching encounters with young, impressionable patients. This encounter was not only an opportunity for the team of students and residents to learn about Emma's rare disorder, it was a teaching moment for the surgeon and his team to learn from Emma and her father about the importance of compassionate communication with their young patient.

Physician Commentary

I have found that often it takes only a minute—literally—to make connections with children and families. Direct eye contact. A smile. A warm greeting. A genuine expression of curiosity of the child's health that day. A touch on the shoulder. Kneeling down to the child and parent level if they are sitting or on a bed. It is not clear from this description whether this attempt to bond was made. But there is more that is needed: permission. The surgeon should have explained to Emma what he was going to do and seek her permission. Give her a role in the teaching process; "can you help me teach these young doctors?" "You are a special girl and these doctors have never met anyone like you before. May I talk to them about you?"

A physician would never enter an adult patient's room and just launch into an exam or procedure without permission. Children should be treated with the same respect. Once children are verbal, permission should be sought. Even if the child is too young to understand, the permission question further establishes a bond with the physician, the child, and the parent(s). This behavior is important in every interaction, but all the more so for children and families with an extensive medical history as in Emma's case. The child may be extra sensitive due to their prior experiences and the families are usually exquisitely tuned to a physician's ability—or inability—to communicate well. Communication is always at the core of physician-patient (or physician-parent) bonding. Without bonding, there is no trust. When there is no trust, there is little chance of a successful therapeutic relationship.

A Sacred Relationship

8

In the Pediatric Intensive Care Unit (PICU), we often see children who are severely neurologically impaired or "devastated" with resultant complex medical issues and limitations with the most fundamental life functions such as communicating, breathing, and eating. The possible causes are myriad: it may be a rare disorder or syndrome, complications from birth, a traumatic injury, secondary to a severe illness in the past, and the list goes on. An awful word I have heard used to describe such a patient is "vegetable"; it makes me cringe that physicians would use such a dehumanizing term. Yet, many would agree that these children have low to no "quality of life." One may even wonder if the child has any meaningful interaction with others, especially their loved ones.

Given their fragility, these children often end up being admitted multiple times a year with all sorts of issues including seizures, pneumonias, urinary tract infections, issues with tracheostomy or gastrostomy tube sites, and electrolyte abnormalities. I cannot even begin to imagine the burden and heartache that the parents and families of these children endure through all the hospitalizations and the arduous care that is required at home. However, physicians are busy in the PICU and it can be easy to lose sight of the humanistic reasons we strived for a career in medicine—to help people, to help children and their families in a time of dire need. Instead, patients often become a laundry list of diagnoses, a checklist of things that need to be done to achieve an ultimate disposition—transfer out of the ICU, discharge home, or even death. So, when a child who is neurologically "devastated" with multiple acute on chronic medical problems is re-admitted many times only to recover to return home to a low "quality of life," this can lead to thoughts and feelings of disappointment or unfulfillment that your hard work is pointless. There was one particular patient encounter I had during my pediatric critical care fellowship training that reconciled such disheartened sentiments and gave me a more enriched perspective of how to care for and love on these children and their families.

Monica, a 4-year-old girl with trisomy 18, holoprosencephaly, and severe facial cleft had been admitted with respiratory failure due to a pneumonia. Upon receiving

© Springer Nature Switzerland AG 2021
A. F. Schrooten, B. P. Markovitz, *Shared Struggles*,
https://doi.org/10.1007/978-3-030-68020-6_8

sign out about this patient for my overnight call, I recognized her as that usual patient with a laundry list of terrible diagnoses and a poor prognosis that we often cared for in the PICU. Her list of diagnoses meant that she had a severely underdeveloped brain; she was blind and could not talk or move without being carried. Her facial cleft left her without any normal facial features. Children born with trisomy 18 and holoprosencephaly rarely survive beyond the first year of life. That Monica had lived to make it to her fourth birthday was remarkable.

Over those 4 years of her life, Monica's parents brought her to the hospital many times with illness after illness to be resuscitated, and she always recovered and was able to return home with her family. However, this time was different. The pneumonia that brought her to the hospital had her in significant respiratory distress and her oxygen levels were dangerously low and dropping further. This was the sickest Monica had ever been and her mother knew it was likely the end. Monica's mother did not want care to be escalated to intubation or chest compressions, and, therefore, she was made "DNR/DNI" which stands for "Do Not Resuscitate/Do Not Intubate." When I am not caught in the hustle and bustle of the ICU and my mind and heart have the time to process what that means—to tell doctors that you do not want your child resuscitated because you love them so much you do not want them to suffer any more—my whole heart aches indescribably.

At 1 am on my overnight shift, the nurse called me to let me know that Monica's oxygen levels were 50% (half of normal and dangerously low) and that she thought Monica would die soon. I quickly came to Monica's room and I explained to her mother that Monica could die at any moment. Her mother's reaction told me that she already knew. She knew her child better than any of us. We asked her if she wanted to hold Monica and she quickly answered "yes." Two nurses and I carried Monica from the bed into her mother's lap. Her mother hugged her daughter tightly and asked the nurse to call her husband, who was at home taking care of the other children, on speakerphone. Monica's father picked up quickly and her mother began quietly crying and quietly repeated the Spanish words *"mi hija…mi hija"* (*my daughter, my daughter*). Monica's father did not say anything but just began crying with Monica's mother over the phone. Soon after their phone call, Monica went into cardiac arrest and passed away.

As Monica's mother tightly hugged her child in the final moments, weeping and crying out "my daughter, my daughter," her pain pierced my heart. In that moment, I saw more clearly that the presence or absence of "meaningful interactions" was not something the physician can truly determine based on a diagnosis or prognosis. Meaning is found in that sacred relationship between the parent and the child, and I now seek to better understand that dynamic. Every child is their parent's entire world and they must be treated that preciously, no matter what. Quality of life has nothing to do with value of life—there is an immeasurable value to every human life.

It is an honor to be able to share in that intimate relationship during a family's time of great need. I believe a parent and child receive better care and also are aware of when their physician compassionately cherishes not only the life of the child, but what the child means to their family. Providing this type of emotionally invested care has actually allowed my heart to reconcile pain that exists for pediatric intensivists in seeing sick children die when we are called into this career to save them, because the families of the children will have known that I truly cared.

Parent Commentary

The measure of quality of life is a sensitive subject for parents of severely disabled children. As the parent of a neurologically impaired child, it stings when I hear that doctors view our children as having a "low" quality of life. Yet, I can also understand how they might feel that way. Before my son was born, and even right after he was born and still in the hospital, if you had asked me, I would not have said a child who would never walk, talk, eat by mouth, or breathe without the assistance of a ventilator could have a good quality of life. My husband and I struggled with the decision of long-term ventilation because we could not imagine a good quality of life for a child who needed a machine to breathe for him 24/7. However, over the 15 years we had with our son, he showed us how wrong we were.

One thing I learned is that assumptions about a child's quality of life should never be based on what you see and experience in the hospital setting. As a parent whose child lived in the Pediatric Intensive Care Unit for most of the first 6 months of his life, certainly being in the hospital with a critically ill child is not a good quality of life for the child or the family. However, most doctors, particularly intensivists, do not get the opportunity to see their patients after they leave the hospital, in their home and community settings. Based on my own experience, a good quality-of-life indicator is having your child be well enough to be home and not in the hospital. Having your child at home opens your eyes to just how much joy and love a child can give and receive notwithstanding their cognitive deficits and physical limitations. As this doctor so beautifully states, it is the relationship we have with our child that gives our child's life value. What our child can or cannot do is not the measure of their worth or quality of life. Our children teach us that a good life is not dependent on a person's ability to walk or talk, or on a person's intelligence, independence, talent, or success. Our children bring into focus what constitutes a good life *for any of us*—feeling loved, feeling safe, and not being in pain. Our neurologically "devastated" children can and do experience these feelings.

What the doctor in this story has come to understand, and what parents want all doctors who care for severely impaired children to understand, is that our child's quality of life cannot be measured based on a snapshot in time, especially when that snapshot is our child in the hospital. Moreover, whether our child has a good quality of life can truly only be determined by us because we experience the whole picture of our child's life.

When our child's health declines and pain and protracted hospital admissions become our child's norm, then, just as Monica's parents had to do, we love our child enough to let them go. Without question, the most agonizing decision a parent will ever have to make is to sign a DNR for their child. We bear this pain because we understand that when our child is suffering, they are no longer living a good life. This decision is not based on our child's abilities, but on a profoundly deep connection and love we have for our child. Our child may have never spoken the words "I love you," but they have shown us what unconditional love looks like, and have taught us the true meaning of a good life.

Physician Commentary

For a long time in the field of pediatric critical care, our most sacred metric of success or failure was a simple, indisputable number: the mortality rate. The better or more advanced our care, the lower the mortality rate. And life was good. Until we realized it was not. Many "survivors" of critical illness suffered disabilities, sometime subtle ones, and the field of studying outcomes—including measures of "quality of life"—has emerged. Outcomes is the new mortality rate. Tools have been developed and validated to measure "quality of life (QOL)," and our work has now shifted to understanding how what we do in the PICU can improve QOL. But QOL is and should not become the new holy grail and this story poignantly illustrates this point.

I could not have stated it better; "Quality of life has nothing to do with value of life—there is an immeasurable value to every human life." As the theme is woven throughout this book, only parents can be the measure of weighing the benefits and burdens of care for their children. Physicians cannot and should never impose their value systems on their patients' families. Our recommendations must always include patient and family values as we partner with them to find the "right" path.

When it is time for the path to end is the most difficult of all such decisions and every child-family-physician triad is different; despite talking about a path, there is no real road map to follow. The map must be found from within, in one's heart. To find that map and follow it to its logical conclusion is always heart rending, and as this physician points out, our hearts can break as well.

Kids Like These

9

We were on our way to the emergency room as I looked back at our oldest daughter, Gwendolyn. She was in her wheelchair, her cheeks were rosy, and her smile wide despite having an oxygen cannula in her nose, and despite the fact that in my hand I was holding her trach tube wrapped in a paper towel. Gwen had pulled her trach out and the hole in her neck where it was supposed to go had closed up too quickly, and we were not able to get the tube back in. This was not the first time Gwen pulled out her trach. However, this time she pulled it out while riding on the school bus and the nurse's aide who traveled with her was unaware of what happened. Gwen had become stealth at yanking out her trach, and on this particular snowy December day, she was all bundled up for school with a scarf wrapped loosely around her neck.

When the nurse took off Gwen's coat after arriving at school, the trach came tumbling out of her scarf. Her teacher called in a panic and asked whether or not to call the ambulance, to which I answered an emphatic "No!" I reassured her that we were on our way and would get there as quickly as we could. Gwen, my husband, and I would then make the three-hour drive to our preferred Children's Hospital.

It had been almost a year since Gwen had her spinal fusion surgery that resulted in a month-long recovery and a tracheostomy before returning home. When the ENT at the Children's Hospital in our town told us she needed a trach to breathe, we were in disbelief because she had passed sleep studies in the past. When he came to talk with me and my husband after the surgery, he pulled out a bell jar graph while uttering "kids like these" phrases, explaining that she would need a tracheostomy at some point in her life, the spinal fusion being her tipping point.

Gwen had already undergone tonsil and adenoid removal, submandibular gland removal, G-tube insertion, three hip osteotomies (two on her right hip and one on her left), and contracted incurable pseudomonas in her lungs from a routine injection of botox. These were just her major medical hurdles. She also endured countless infections, fevers, seizures, ER trips, specialist appointments, and therapy appointments. But it was the diagnostic phrase "kids like these" and the tracheostomy that broke me open.

© Springer Nature Switzerland AG 2021
A. F. Schrooten, B. P. Markovitz, *Shared Struggles*,
https://doi.org/10.1007/978-3-030-68020-6_9

After her spinal fusion surgery and a week into her recovery from the insertion of the trach, a medicine dosing error was discovered. As Gwen was trying to recover from the spinal fusion surgery, she was getting too much valium, and this caused her to have continual apnea episodes. In turn, she was having trouble getting off oxygen since her surgery. These setbacks caused everyone on the medical team, including me, to agree that a tracheostomy was the appropriate next step to get Gwen home.

We asked for a meeting with Gwen's medical team and nurse management. We were reassured that there was no concrete evidence of a correlation between the dosing error and Gwen's need for a trach and, again, were told, "kids like these" would always eventually need a trach.

Devastated and disheartened, we brought Gwen home just after Christmas. It was our first Christmas spent in the hospital, and we learned that there are far too many children who spend the holidays in the hospital. Because of the trach, Gwen lost her ability to vocalize and that was a significant loss for us, especially because she did not talk. Despite our home health nurse's assurance that, with time, Gwen would be able to use a special cap to produce sounds, we felt defeated. Within a matter of days after coming home from the hospital, Gwen, who had very little hand dexterity, hooked her pinkie around her trach and yanked it out. The first time we attributed it to an accident, but as time went on, it became very apparent this was very much a deliberate act.

At her follow-up appointment with the ENT, I asked if it was possible she might no longer need the trach, having fully recovered from her surgery. He emphasized again "kids like these" and would not entertain the possibility of permanently removing the trach.

After leaving his office, I knew we had to do better. I began to research a Children's Hospital that was a three-hour drive from our home. I read on their website about the pediatric otorhinolaryngology program. As a teaching hospital, the approach to complex pediatric airways was to treat each child as an individual. My husband and I agreed it was time for a second opinion. However, I did not get a chance to make an appointment before Gwen gave us the opportunity to take a risk and drive to this other hospital because she was unexpectedly trach-less.

When arrived at the emergency department, the first major difference from our local hospital was the intake. Never before had an intake nurse looked at me as the expert and asked how I felt Gwen was doing without her trach before rushing us back. In a matter of minutes, the chief doctor from the pediatric otorhinolaryngology team was at Gwen's bedside, "This must be the super hero I've been hearing about." Gwen started to giggle. He spoke to Gwen, "You are quite the mastermind Gwen. I've heard this has become quite the trick you've mastered, dislodging your trach."

He then looked at me. "How do you feel she is doing without the trach?"

"Well, she's not in distress and she's happy." I replied.

He said the only way the trach would be going back in would be with surgery. I remember looking at him as he looked over Gwen. There was a sense of true compassion. He told us, "I'd like to admit her for twenty-four hours to see how she does without oxygen and the trach. But as far as I can see now, she does not need to have it reinserted." Before he left the room, he took Gwen's hand in his and told her, "You are one amazing kiddo."

We were transferred to the floor for our overnight stay. Settled in bed, Gwen began to laugh. In fact, she was so pleased to hear her own voice again, her laughter continued. She laughed through her blood draws, through her vitals being taken, through the entire night. I was so sleep deprived and every time I told her to quiet down, she laughed even harder. She laughed so hard she was holding her breath and set off her low oxygen alarm. Each time the nurse came in, she was surprised that Gwen was still laughing.

The following morning, the doctor stopped in to look at Gwen's chart and examine her. He asked me how her night went. Her stoma was nearly completely closed by now and I told him that she had rediscovered her voice and was sharing laughs with all of us. He told us that he doubted Gwen ever needed a tracheostomy based on her history and what he observed. He acknowledged that some doctors are quick to make judgments and lump kids into groups and treatment plans based on a diagnosis or set of problems. He asked us to follow-up in 6 months and handed me Gwen's discharge paperwork. He then pulled a small box wrapped with a gold ribbon out of his pocket, "I saved this for you, Gwen. Maybe you can hang it on your Christmas tree." When we got home that evening, we unwrapped the box. Inside was a clean trach made into an ornament that was signed to the *Most Incredible Gwendolyn.*

This doctor is an accomplished expert in his field. Yet, it is not his many accolades that sets him apart, it is his compassion, his willingness to see the parents as the experts of their child, and his ability to listen to his patients. He sees "kids like these" as more than a predetermined outcome based on a bell graph. He approaches each child as a unique individual and looks to the child—not the diagnosis—for guidance on how best to proceed for that child. His compassion and willingness to take the time for meaningful communication meant Gwen regained her own voice. It also meant we as her parents felt heard and valued. His compassion gave us all another chance to trust the medical system and move forward with hope.

Parent Commentary

Reading this story makes me think of the opportunities given to our typical, healthy children. Parents of healthy children see their child's potential and do everything they can to maximize it. They spend their time and money on club sports, lessons, camps, tutors, and the list goes on. A typical, healthy child is given the opportunity to excel and be the exception—the "star" player, musician, or student. A disabled, medically complex child deserves the same opportunity to be the stand out, the exception when it comes to the opportunities and challenges they are presented with.

The first ENT did not appear to present the tracheostomy as the best option for Gwen, rather, he presented it as the only option. It does not seem that he took into consideration that Gwen was doing well without a trach before surgery and had passed multiple sleep studies in the past. It is very possible that Gwen needed a trach to get her through recovery from spinal fusion surgery. However, the better approach would have been to discuss the trach as a temporary intervention with the option to have it removed following another sleep study.

The second ENT had the advantage of seeing Gwen doing well without the trach. This afforded him and Gwen's parents the option to "wait and see" before making any decisions regarding re-inserting the trach. This doctor also allowed Gwen to guide the decision, rather than make the decision based on the purported norm for children with similar conditions and diagnoses as Gwen. He compassionately gave Gwen the opportunity and time to show what she was capable of without the trach.

Decisions regarding interventions for our medically complex children should be presented on an individual patient-by-patient basis and not based on statistics or probabilities looking at a group of similarly diagnosed patients. Our children should be given the opportunity to write their own story. The fact is, it is not likely that our typical kid will sign a multi-million dollar contract with the NFL, play a solo at Carnegie Hall, or win the Nobel Peace Prize. However, we do not tell them they are just one of the "average" kids, so do not bother trying. Likewise, our disabled, medically complex children should not be grouped together and given predetermined outcomes. Every child deserves the chance to be the stand out—the exception—within the context of their own unique opportunities and challenges.

Physician Commentary

As a physician, I cannot count the number of times a patient has surprised me, "beating the odds" and proving our statistical approach to patient care as woefully inadequate. I would venture to say that there is NO diagnosis in Pediatrics that mandates any particular treatment or non-treatment, except, sadly, the diagnosis of death itself. Every patient is their own textbook. Even conditions that we understand—or think we do—at the molecular level (sickle cell disease comes to mind—a single gene defect), have a wide variety of phenotypes or clinical presentations. Some children with a particular diagnosis need extraordinary levels of care, others, not so much. The patient tells us what they need.

The other lesson from this story is that children change. Even those with defined diagnoses that the textbooks (presumably) tell us will inexorably progress with loss of function. Some children with significant genetic abnormalities will never be "normal," but they can achieve a meaningful (defined by them and their families, not physicians) level of quality of life and powerful relationships over time. It is hard to generalize here since some children have "static" injuries, such as birth asphyxia, whereas others have progressive genetic diseases. Nevertheless, no patient is a statistic and they—with their families and care providers as partners—should chart each course individually.

A Smile Worth Saving

10

We call our son Anthony our "ray of sunshine" because he is always happy. Anthony has spastic quadriplegic cerebral palsy and a profound developmental disability. He is wheelchair dependent, does not speak, and is fed through a gastrostomy-jejunostomy (GJ) feeding tube. In spite of his significant disability, he is a happy, healthy kid who is famous for his smile.

Early one morning as I was getting Anthony ready for school, I could tell he was not his usual happy self. He was lethargic and his muscle tone was low, which is unusual for him because he has spastic cerebral palsy. I figured he was coming down with something and decided to keep him home from school. As part of his routine morning care, I went to flush his feeding tube. When I opened the GJ port, blood started draining back out of the tube, and, based on the amount of blood that was coming out, it was obvious whatever was going on was serious. I decided the safest thing to do was call 9-1-1.

The ambulance showed up within minutes, and when the EMTs walked into our house, one of them fainted when he saw all the blood that had come out of Anthony's feeding tube. This required a second ambulance to be called! One ambulance took off with the EMT; the other ambulance took Anthony to the emergency department. We got to the hospital around 7:30 am.

In the emergency department, they took Anthony's vital signs and started an IV. At this point, Anthony's heart rate was 130. His baseline heart rate runs high, but this was higher than usual. All his lab work came back normal and his vital signs were stable, except for his elevated heart rate. The emergency department attending called Anthony's gastroenterologist who advised us to increase one of Anthony's medications and follow-up with him in the office later in the week. When the attending told us what the gastroenterologist suggested, I was not at all comfortable with the plan. There was no way I was going to take Anthony home with blood coming out of his GJ-tube. He was sick and I knew something was wrong.

The attending asked me how much blood were we talking about. I told her, "As much as you want. Just open the tube and it drains blood." I unplugged the GJ-tube port and blood came pouring out. Obviously surprised, the doctor said, "OK, that's

© Springer Nature Switzerland AG 2021
A. F. Schrooten, B. P. Markovitz, *Shared Struggles*,
https://doi.org/10.1007/978-3-030-68020-6_10

enough, I get the point." She asked me, "Did the resident see this?" I told her, "No," but that I had explained to him what was going on. "Well, seeing is believing," she said. Even though I told the nurse and the resident that a significant amount of blood was coming out of Anthony's GJ-tube, neither one of them checked the tube to assess what was going on. After seeing the blood, the attending ordered abdominal X-rays and a surgical consultation. The X-ray was unremarkable, but Anthony was obviously getting worse as the day went on. His heart rate was now in the 150s. His other vital signs remained stable.

The on-call surgeon came to see Anthony. He was an older gentleman who seemed inconvenienced to be there. His examination of Anthony consisted of pressing on his stomach a few times, after which he told the attending, "This is not a surgical matter." He then walked out of the room without acknowledging or addressing me or my husband.

The attending wanted to admit Anthony for observation; however, I felt Anthony needed more than observation. I am a nurse and, based on my experience, I thought he might have a bowel obstruction, perforated bowel, or necrotic bowel. All serious issues. None of the doctors felt Anthony had any of these things, but I was not convinced. He was getting sicker and sicker by the hour. He was in obvious pain and he was still bleeding from his feeding tube. His heart rate was climbing and was now over 160.

Although Anthony cannot talk, his facial expressions and heart rate told me he was in pain. I told the emergency department staff repeatedly that something was seriously wrong, but no one felt the same sense of urgency that I did. They did not know our happy boy—they only saw a child who was severely disabled.

Before admitting him, a doctor from the medical floor came down to the emergency department to see Anthony. By this time, Anthony's heart rate was over 180. I quickly explained what was going on with Anthony and this doctor actually listened to me. I heard him tell both the attending and resident that Anthony was too unstable to go to the regular floor. Finally, they began to understand that something serious was going on and ordered an abdominal CT scan. From the look on the resident's face when he came to give us the results, we knew it did not look good. The surgeon was called back in. After seeing the CT scan, he brought us to a small conference room and sat us down to go over our options. Nothing could have prepared us for what he had to say.

Based on Anthony's symptoms and the CT scan, it appeared Anthony had diffuse damage throughout his intestinal tract. The surgeon said there was not a single area that he could "fix." Usually in cases of obstruction, perforation, or necrosis, the damaged part of the bowel can be removed. However, in Anthony's case, the CT scan showed swelling and white spots throughout his entire intestine, which appeared to be massive tissue damage. There was also fluid, presumably blood, in his peritoneal cavity. The surgeon told us he could do an exploratory surgery but it was unlikely he would be able to repair this type of damage. The surgeon gave us two options: do the surgery or "let nature take its course." The surgeon asked, "Do you really want to put a kid like Anthony through this major surgery?" He explained that Anthony was very sick and likely would not tolerate the surgery well. He did not believe the outcome would be good. After the surgery, Anthony would have a long and complicated post-operative course. He would likely have an infection, which could easily lead to a downward spiral. Did we really want to put him through this?

We got the distinct feeling we were being discouraged from doing the surgery. It was obvious that the surgeon did not want to operate on Anthony. We felt that he did not view Anthony as having a good quality of life because of his severe disabilities. The surgeon did not know that Anthony was the happiest kid in the world when he was feeling well. He did not appreciate that Anthony is an important part of a loving family, that he has a great quality of life, and he has many friends at school and in his community. We felt the surgeon was giving us the worst-case scenario only. Regardless, the prognosis we were given was very grim and we were heartbroken.

Despite the surgeon's efforts to discourage us from the surgery, my husband and I both agreed to an exploratory surgery. It was an easy decision for us. We needed to know exactly what we were dealing with and the only sure way of knowing was to open him up. We were also asked about a do-not-resuscitate order. We made it clear we wanted everything done for Anthony until we had reason to think otherwise.

Anthony was finally taken to the operating room at 9:45 pm that night. My husband and I sat in the surgical waiting area, both feeling numb. Everything happened so quickly. I was having a typical morning getting the kids up and off to school. Just hours later, one of our boys was on death's door. It just seemed unreal. What would we do without Anthony? How would we tell his brothers? While I wanted to know what was wrong with Anthony, I dreaded meeting with the surgeon after the surgery. I was afraid to hear bad news.

The surgery took about 3 hours. When the surgeon came out to find us, we were the only people left in the waiting room. As he walked across the room, he said, "He's OK" before he even got to us. The surgeon explained that most of the "necrosis" he had seen on the CT scan was actually air in Anthony's bowel. He had developed a rare complication from the GJ-tube. His small intestine wrapped around the tube and caused a kink in his bowel, this cut off the blood supply to the intestine around the GJ-tube. That segment of his bowel was necrotic—dead from lack of blood flow. The surgeon removed about one-fourth of Anthony's small intestine and sutured the ends of the healthy intestine back together.

With a situation like Anthony's, the longer it takes for a patient to get to surgery, the more the intestine dies. Had we waited much longer—or done nothing at all, Anthony surely would have died in a very short time. The surgeon's efforts to discourage us from going through with the surgery conveyed the message that Anthony's life was not worth saving because of his severe disability. Individuals with disabilities are commonly viewed as a burden to their families and to society. Too often, little value is placed on their lives. I am confident that if Anthony had been a typical child, he would have been taken to the operating room right away. Instead, he waited over 12 hours before receiving the proper treatment. This delay made his condition worse and his surgery more complicated, and it nearly cost him his life. When we went to see Anthony in the postoperative area after surgery, the nurse caring for him looked at us and said, "Good job advocating for your son."

Parent Commentary

Sadly, what this family experienced with the surgeon is not uncommon for families of severely disabled children. I have experienced my share of doctors who viewed my son's life as "less than" when it came to the care and treatment he received. While you never hear those words, they come across loud and clear in the first interaction with the doctor and how they treat your child. I cannot count the number of times a doctor walked in an exam or hospital room and talked to me as if my son was invisible. Not so much as a "hello" was spoken to him. Humans are social beings and we want to engage with people. Unfortunately, most people only know how to engage through spoken conversation, and when your patient is disabled and nonverbal, it takes exceptional patience and powers of observation to connect and communicate with them. More importantly, it takes a desire to *want* to communicate with them.

Beyond the failure to acknowledge our child's presence, is the often-felt resistance to medically treat our child the same they would a non-disabled, communicative child—like the family in this story experienced. That being said, having had my own child cared for by many doctors and at different institutions, I believe how our child is treated can vary greatly depending on how many severely disabled patients a doctor sees and how long-standing the patient-doctor relationship is. Those doctors whose practice includes caring for a large population of severely disabled children see our children over the course of many years, they see the relationships they have with their parents, and they hear about the relationships they have with their families and communities. Our children, by their very existence, teach these doctors (and so many others) that their life has tremendous quality and value. (This is not to say that *only* those doctors who regularly care for severely disabled children provide compassionate and non-disparate care.)

It is through the strong and relentless advocating by parents like Anthony's that we educate and open the eyes of those who provide care to our children and ensure that they receive the same level of treatment, care, and compassion that would be extended to any other child, regardless of "ability."

Physician Commentary

This is a near tragedy, and I must agree that all too often, physicians who do not know a patient and their family have an implicit bias that children with significant disabilities should not have the same level of aggressive medical care immediately offered to "normal" children. I am reassured that parents of these children, as this child's parents did, learn to advocate and help the health care professionals put such acute situations in perspective. In addition, most of these children have a primary physician who knows the child and family and can also be an ally in advocacy for the child.

I do want to distinguish between children with "static"—or nonprogressive—conditions, compared to those with "progressive" diseases. Cerebral palsy, or static encephalopathy, is, by definition, a static and nonprogressive condition. These children certainly have limitations, sometimes severe, but they can, as Anthony in this story, have a highly meaningful quality of life by anyone's view. However, there are conditions that are progressive, associated with loss of functioning over time, and these situations are extremely difficult for parents and physicians to navigate when acute illnesses occur. These children will ultimately succumb to their disease, and decisions do need to be made when life-threatening crises occur about what the "right" thing to do is for the child. This is not such a situation, in my opinion.

One other comment is relevant in this situation. Parents can find advocating for their children in these situations exhausting. They must thread the needle of speaking up for their child, while not antagonizing the health care team with what can be perceived as being overly strident and even hostile. How did this family speak up for Anthony when they perceived he was essentially being discriminated against because of his disability? Were they polite and respectful? Did they express outrage that Anthony was being minimized? Alas, parents such as Anthony's must be polite, respectful, and deferential to the medical "authority" held by the physicians and still find a way to speak for their child who cannot speak for him or herself. It is not fair, but it is reality. My fellow physicians, first seek to understand. Put yourself in your patients' parents' shoes. Wear their glasses. The world can and should look differently.

Part II

Trust

Trust is the glue of life. It's the most essential ingredient in effective communication. It's the foundational principle that holds all relationships. –Stephen R. Covey

Team Harlie

11

For an anesthesiologist, one of our most critical pieces of information is the ever-present beep of the pulse oximeter. The tone—how high or low pitched it is—tells us how much oxygen our patient's blood is carrying to the tissues of their body: their brain, their kidneys, and their heart. We can know what is going on without ever taking our eyes off of our patient—and at midnight, staring down at Harlie, I knew things were not going well.

On a busy call night, after just finishing an emergent case for a devastatingly sick premature baby, our team was called to the ICU to assist in an emergent reintubation. In the middle of the night, this is never good. Our ICU doctors are very skilled at placing breathing tubes for patients who cannot breathe on their own, so when they call for anesthesia assistance, it usually indicates a very difficult intubation or a very complicated patient. Harlie was both.

I got a quick signout from the ICU doctor on call, prepped the operating room for every possible contingency, had every tool and trick available for a difficult airway, and scurried up to Harlie's bedside to meet her.

We are trained to make first impressions, and this was mine: Harlie was tired, struggling to breathe despite a BiPAP mask and machine that was assisting her every breath. Her face was dysmorphic—different—her bone structure was not typical and portended a challenging airway. Her oxygen saturation was low—this I had to *see* because outside of the OR or a code blue, the monitors typically do not audibly beep. But as I stood at Harlie's bedside and looked around the room, it was the shirts that struck me. Harlie's family was wearing matching t-shirts of support for her. *THIS* alerted me to how much this family had been through and how tightly they had joined together to love and support Harlie and one another. *THIS* was the clue I needed to understand how tenuous Harlie's situation was, and looking around the room at the faces of her worried surgeons, I knew we did not have a lot of time, and I knew this was not going to be easy. This was all ascertained within the first 30 seconds of entering Harlie's room.

© Springer Nature Switzerland AG 2021
A. F. Schrooten, B. P. Markovitz, *Shared Struggles*,
https://doi.org/10.1007/978-3-030-68020-6_11

Upon further inquiry, I learned that Harlie did not just have a difficult airway; she also had a complex cardiac condition that made this reintubation anything but commonplace. She was born with transposition of the great arteries with a hypoplastic right ventricle—this had been surgically addressed 7 years prior, leaving her with a single ventricle pumping blood to her body and blood flowing passively to her lungs through a conduit, called a Fontan, that also allowed blood to bypass her lungs if the pressure in them became too high. Because of this physiology, she was likely to have desaturation episodes and be very slow to recover from them. Additionally, it also predisposed her to venous congestion, such that bleeding in her airway would be more likely and more pronounced. I told her mother, while hurriedly pushing Harlie's hospital bed toward the OR doors, trying my best not to appear rushed: "I'm going to take care of her like she's my own until I give her back to you." I meant every word.

There was literally no room for error in this situation. Harlie laid on the operating room table, still on her BiPAP machine, and we knew that we had precious little time between removing her from this support and securing her airway with a breathing tube. Given her clinical status and her heart condition, her oxygen saturation would plummet without the support she was currently receiving and be very slow to recover, and any bleeding in her airway during the attempt at intubation would be significant. Further complicating our plans, she needed a nasal intubation, as it would be more stable and she was a feisty little girl who was likely to pull out a breathing tube placed in the mouth. Given the difficulty of intubation and the precarious situation an inadvertent extubation would produce, every member of the team was on the same page. Surrounding the bedside, we took a pause to discuss the plan—and then plans B, C, and D.

After inducing general anesthesia through a mask, we removed the mask and placed a flexible fiber-optic camera into her nose. The amount of airway swelling was immense, and there were no recognizable structures seen on the screen to anyone in the room. This was going to be a difficult approach, even in the best of circumstances with ample time, and we did not have ample time. We had seconds. As soon as the breathing tube was introduced, we also encountered bleeding, which further complicated our approach. We removed the scope and resumed breathing for Harlie through the mask, but as expected, her oxygen saturation dropped and was not coming all the way back up. The beeps dropped in tone and never rose to the higher pitch where we had started.

The team worked seamlessly, but it was clear that plan A would not be successful; we could not place a breathing tube through the nose and we had precious few opportunities remaining. The ear, nose, and throat (ENT) surgeons were also unable to place a breathing tube through the mouth. After their attempt, the pitch of the beeping fell again, and again did not rise back to her new lower baseline. We were still able to mask ventilate in between attempts, but it was becoming more difficult and it was clear to all in the room that we were out of chances and a next attempt could lead to tragedy.

"Does anyone in this room see any other way than a tracheostomy to secure her airway?" I asked. No one did, so we prepped her neck for a surgical airway. I am not sure I can describe the feeling of making the call to convert to an emergent surgical airway. The sentiment is somewhere between desperation and surrender, and it is never, ever a decision made lightly or without a tangible understanding of the risk-benefit ratio. We decided to trach Harlie that night because we thought she would die if we did not. This was not her first trach either—she had been down this road before and recovered, so it was an even weightier decision this time. The low pitch of the beeping constantly reminded us of the dire situation we currently were in.

Ultimately, a tracheostomy was performed and we were able to return Harlie to the ICU for further care. Hours had seemed like moments, but I was finally able to find Harlie's mother and update her on what had happened. She was in a small side room of the ICU. These rooms are available for families at all hours—sometimes a meeting area, sometimes a hiding place, and sometimes just a place for a family to gather for a meal away from the ubiquitous medical reminders of current circumstance. But tonight, it was decidedly a waiting room and to Harlie's mother, I assume, the hours had felt like days.

I spent a long time talking with Harlie's mother—we were away far longer than anticipated and learning that her mother assumed that this meant Harlie had not made it humbled me in a way nothing else could. I was sad to have brought Harlie back with a tracheostomy, especially given it was a thing she and her family had already overcome once before. But at the same time, I was so grateful to be bringing back a live child, and those dual feelings were shared by her mother as well.

The next morning, I ventured to Harlie's bedside again. That combination of relief and sadness was palpable and honest. We took a couple of selfies that Harlie's mother said she would send my way and I wished them the very best.

I never got those pictures.

Nearly 2 years later, I finally heard from Harlie's mother. I was at home watching TV with my family when the e-mail came in and, in short, it took my breath away. I had thought about them often and always assumed that I had never heard from her because it was a bad night they just wanted to forget. I think I had always hoped this and respected it. As I finally saw those pictures and read the account of everything they had been through over the past 2 years—the complications and setbacks—everything in my world came into focus on this one little girl and this one night on call.

I saw Harlie and her parents when they returned to our hospital after being away so long and was struck by how much Harlie had grown and how she absolutely exuded life and resilience. In many respects, given I had only met her in a time of crisis, I was essentially meeting her for the first time. She was feisty indeed and to be honest, I was struck by how full of joy she was. After all she had been through—all of the procedures, tests, hospitalizations—she was, after all, still a little girl.

I later met the family at a team meeting, where it was openly discussed how they could move forward, and I was awestruck by the tenacious optimism and pragmatism of her parents. I could see where Harlie got her joyful nature and was grateful to get to know them better. Just before leaving to head back home that evening, after getting to spend additional time with Harlie and her family, I was given 2 years of Christmas cards that had never been sent and a "Team Harlie" t-shirt. *THAT* shirt—the one that brought the situation into focus 2 years prior—was now in my hands. I was officially on Team Harlie and I am still not sure the family realizes how much that meant to me.

I guess the real question is how things like this change you as a physician, and I think the truth is that it is complicated and cumulative. I have learned to try to keep my ego out of medical outcomes and relationships far more—it is simply not about me. Bad results are often the result of bad circumstances and may even be the best result possible. Good results are often the result of blind luck and teamwork. In medicine, it is so easy to focus on our deficits, and it is a conscious act to bring a more fair focus on the work we perform. Anesthesiologists are notoriously meticulous and controlling—it helps us do our job. But it also predisposes us to taking bad outcomes very personally, even the aspects of which we have absolutely no control.

As anesthesiologists, we have fewer opportunities than most physicians to develop long-standing or deep relationships with patients and families, so when they happen, they are precious and notable. I would have understood if, given the turn of events, this family had never wanted to see me again. I would have understood if they requested different providers going forward, whether from a lack of confidence, superstition, or simply the reminder of that night. But instead, they reached out, asked me to care for their child again and welcomed me onto Team Harlie! It is a profound privilege to be entrusted with the care of another's child but exponentially more so in a situation such as this. And for me, there is no greater honor than the opportunity to care for Harlie again.

Parent Commentary

There is much written about what factors are instrumental in establishing trust between a patient (or parent of a patient) and a doctor. In this story, the doctor seemed surprised that Harlie's parents reconnected with her after a less than ideal outcome for Harlie that this doctor played a role in. However, from a parent's perspective, it is easy to understand where this trust came from. While Harlie's parents may not have known it at the time, this doctor immediately appreciated the impact Harlie had on her family and all that they had been through when she took notice of the "Team Harlie" t-shirts everyone was wearing. And while the doctor may have not known it at the time, I think it is fair to say that she joined "Team Harlie" the moment she wheeled Harlie back to the operating room, as I cannot think of anything more comforting and reassuring than being told by your child's doctor that she will care for your child like she is her own.

After Harlie came out of surgery, this doctor spent time with Harlie's mother. It was late and things had not gone as planned. It would not have been unreasonable for this doctor to spend only as much time needed to convey what happened in the operating room and continue the conversation the next morning. However, she sat down with Harlie's mother, she explained what happened, and she was moved by Harlie's mother's worry and fear that her daughter had died. She was sad that Harlie had to be re-trached. When a doctor is genuinely affected by your child's outcome, this honesty and transparency comes through. Knowing that a doctor is invested in your child strengthens a parent's trust.

This doctor also kept the lines of communication open. She provided Harlie's mother with her email and gave her permission to stay in touch and let her know how Harlie was doing. She wanted to support this family after they left the hospital.

There are many factors that contribute to a trusting relationship with our child's doctor. As was so well displayed by the doctor in this story, trust is created when doctors notice us and our child and appreciate what we have been through; when they care for our child as their own; when they spend time with us and are honest, genuine, and transparent; and when they are accessible and provide us with their contact information and respond to our emails and phone calls.

Harlie's mother trusted this doctor, and, because of this trust, she had no reservations about putting Harlie's care in her hands again. When we trust our child's doctor, we are better able to deal with the difficult, unexpected, and unwanted outcomes for our child.

Physician Commentary

Many physicians (and perhaps the lay public) view anesthesiologists as technicians. They put you to sleep and wake you up. There is rarely any kind of therapeutic relationship formed. How wrong this view is. Pediatric anesthesiologists must, even in elective situations, meet a child and their parents and within minutes establish a trusting bond that allows parents to hand over the thing in this world that means the most to them—their child. Parents must trust this physician to put their child into a coma (we call it sleep, but it is truly a medically induced coma), protect and watch over them like a mother hawk during the operation, and then return them to their baseline level of consciousness safely. The physician in this story, in the heat of a dire emergency, said the words that this mother needed to hear to establish that trust, almost in a heartbeat.

This physician further defined the unique role of the pediatric anesthesiologist in securing the family's trust by talking to them extensively immediately after the procedure. The truth was provided without sugar coating. There was no defensiveness or blaming. No doubt this transparency cemented the bond with this family. A bond that lasted for years, from one encounter.

This message of bonding and trust is generalizable to all physicians who care for children. Speak the truth, with compassion, hope, and empathy, and you will at least be heard and begin the journey of trust that is vital to both parent and physician for the best outcomes possible.

Best Laid Plans 12

Keyan was admitted to our Children's Hospital in early December for high fever, pneumonia, and c-diff. The hospital staff did their best to bring holiday cheer to their young patients—colorful stockings hung from the nurses' station and miniature Christmas trees brightened patient rooms. Nevertheless, the hospital was the last place any family wanted to be this time of the year. With Christmas Day fast approaching, we were doing everything we could think of to get Keyan home from the hospital.

When Keyan is in the hospital, I usually stay with her the entire time, never leaving the hospital. However, in this particular admission, we made arrangements for one of Keyan's home health nurses to sit with her for the afternoon and evening because I needed to finish up shopping and take care of other holiday preparations.

For 3 days leading up to that day, I talked with every doctor, nurse, therapist, child life specialist, and probably even housekeeping. I prepared them ahead of time that I would be gone for a portion of the day. As a team, we talked through my expectations for Keyan while I was gone. I reiterated over and over that they please only do Keyan's routine care with no changes unless they discussed it with me ahead of time.

Keyan is one of quadruplets born premature at 27 weeks. Her health issues include chronic lung disease and a non-functioning gastrointestinal system that requires she receive all her nutrition intravenously through a broviac central line. Keyan's daily care consists of multiple medications, chest percussion therapy to keep her lungs clear, central line care, and monitoring of her continuous tube feedings. Keyan is medically complicated and a seemingly simple change can have a negative domino effect. It is important to know her history and how she reacts to changes. A medical chart may give her healthcare team data but it cannot give them the details that only the parent of a medically fragile child knows based on years of experience.

Before leaving the hospital, both my husband and I left our contact information in case they needed to reach us for anything. I felt comfortable that I had covered all my bases. When I returned to the hospital for the night, I walked into Keyan's room

© Springer Nature Switzerland AG 2021
A. F. Schrooten, B. P. Markovitz, *Shared Struggles*,
https://doi.org/10.1007/978-3-030-68020-6_12

and found her in major distress. Her heart rate had skyrocketed, she was crying because of abdominal pain, and she was gagging and retching nonstop. Things had clearly taken a turn for the worse during the time I was gone.

I barraged Keyan's home health nurse with questions. I tracked down the hospital nurses and questioned them. I desperately tried to put the missing pieces together. Everyone was working to "put out the fires" and find relief for Keyan. No one could give me any indication of why she was in distress. Her central line seemed intact. Her tube feeding was set to the proper rate. She had received all of her usual medications. I knew there was always the possibility this could be an out of the ordinary episode, but my instincts told me something had been changed with Keyan's routine care while I was gone. My hopes of having her home for Christmas faded as the night progressed.

Not long after I returned to the hospital, a nurse walked into Keyan's room and said she had Keyan's next dose of oral antibiotic to give her. I froze. When I left earlier that day, she was not on any oral antibiotics. I took a deep breath and calmly asked her what she was talking about. She said the hospitalist rounded while I was gone and switched Keyan's antibiotic from IV to oral. He ordered a loading oral dose shortly after I left and she was due for another dose.

I could not believe what I was hearing. I was so careful to make sure everyone knew what Keyan's medication and care routine was. I knew Keyan reacts terribly to the oral form of this particular antibiotic. It wreaks havoc on her gastrointestinal system. She can tolerate it through her central line if it is run very slowly and she is pre-treated with antihistamines.

Keyan spent so much time inpatient at our Children's Hospital that the staff knew her well. They also knew me and trusted and respected my knowledge of Keyan's complicated medical issues. The hospitalist who made the change in the antibiotic was a new doctor at the hospital. He did not know Keyan or me. Earlier in the week, this doctor and I had gone round and round about other matters involving Keyan's medical care. I explained to him that while her routine care plan may not always make sense medically, I know my daughter and she does not do anything by the book.

Why had he changed it? Why was not I called? Why did not someone think to question his decision?

I was angry and frustrated. It may appear to be a minor decision in the doctor's eyes, but it was going to have major repercussions for our daughter. I was devastated. I knew these complications would keep her in the hospital over the holidays. Even more, it meant unnecessary suffering for Keyan. I blamed myself for not being there to prevent the medication change. But I also believed had the hospitalist given me the respect I deserved as Keyan's mother and advocate, the mistake would not have happened.

It is frustrating and exhausting to feel trapped at the hospital with your sick and medically complex child because you are afraid of what might happen if you leave. Keyan did indeed spend Christmas in the hospital that year. We made the best of it, but I wondered if it could have been different if the doctor and medical team had only listened to me.

Parent Commentary

I believe most parents of a medically complex child who spend time in and out of the hospital will tell you that there are those doctors who will always listen to us and those doctors who will not. The doctors who recognize us as the expert when it comes to our child are usually those who have seen us in action, time and time again through admission after admission. The doctors who do not listen to us are generally those who are new to us. They do not know our child, they do not know us, and they have not had a lot of experience with medically complex kids.

There are many times when our child is admitted to the hospital for a recurring issue that we have an idea of what the problem is and what needs to be done to resolve it. We bring our child to the hospital not because we do not know what the issue is, but because we do not have the resources to resolve the problem at home. We can be stubborn, impatient, and demanding, but I also believe that more times than not, we know what we are talking about and are usually correct.

There are also those times when we do not know what is going on with our child, and for many of us, our child is unable to verbalize what they are feeling or what hurts. We are at a loss, but we can still read our child better than a doctor who does not know our child or their baseline. We know something is wrong, and, based on our experience, we have an idea of what the medical team should be focusing on. We convey our theory of what is going on and we become frustrated when our ideas are brushed off and not considered. However, I have also learned that I can be wrong—that what I insist is this admission's issue with my child is not the case. I have learned to accept that while I am the expert when it comes to my child, the doctors caring for my child have expertise too, and I must be open to listen to what they have to say.

It really all comes down to trust. If a parent feels that the doctor caring for their child trusts the parent's expertise, then it is much easier for the parent to trust the doctor when his or her opinion of what the issue might be does not align with the parent's. A doctor gains a parent's trust when they show genuine respect for the parent's opinions, suggestions, and ideas and take the time to thoughtfully explain why they disagree or have a different opinion or plan of care.

This story did not involve a situation where Keyan's mother was asking the medical team to consider her care requests surrounding an unknown issue. It was not a situation where deferral to the expertise of the doctor was necessary. It was a request involving routine care of an exceptionally medically complex child. We do not know the doctor's reasoning behind changing the route of administering Keyan's antibiotic. Being new and not knowing Keyan well, he probably had no reason to expect that this simple change would result in such a negative outcome for Keyan. However, being new and not knowing Keyan well is the very reason he should have honored her mother's request to keep Keyan's routine care the status quo during her short absence.

Physician Commentary

This is clearly a case of miscommunication or lack of communication between a physician and a parent. As more and more of our inpatients have complex medical problems, pediatricians in training usually learn early on which patients' parents are highly knowledgeable and involved. We learn which parents want to be called, day or night about any changes in their child. But this assumes the child is under our care to start with.

Physicians who are hospital-based, such as intensivists or hospitalists, only work in the hospital and usually rotate their "service" duties. A physician may care for a child for a week and then hand off the care to another physician. Usually these handoffs are thorough and include issues about the patients' families. We also often have separate doctors "in house" at night. They are there to address changes in patients and admit new ones. They usually do not go around at night and make big changes in plans for the patients they are covering. All of this is to say that physicians can be responsible for dozens of patients and the handoff process is not fool proof. It is pure speculation to wonder why this physician made a change in Keyan's treatment without calling the mother or father. One also wonders why this mother did not talk to the covering physician before the parents left to make sure he knew of their strong wishes. Yes, perhaps the nurses should have "run cover" and made sure this physician knew the situation, but maybe that expectation also slipped through a crack.

The flip side of this story is the glass half-full view. It seems like this family—except for this instance—does have a strong and trusting relationship with the team at this hospital, and the parents' wisdom and expertise about Keyan is listened to and heeded regularly. Perhaps because that is the normative relationship this family has, this incident stands out in their minds as so terribly problematic. Trust, however, takes a lot of time and effort to build, yet it can be lost in an instant.

If We Are Paying Attention

13

I met Bryan and his mom, Olivia, when I was a pediatric resident. I may have met them as an intern, but Bryan spent a lot more time in the hospital during my senior years, and that is the time I remember him best. Bryan was born with severe hydranencephaly. We joked that he was a thin rim of brain cells away from anencephaly. Not particularly professional or kind, but that is the reality. As far as I could tell, Bryan had no appreciable interaction with the outside world. I was a second-year resident and thought I knew it all. In my early training, it was not unusual to spend 120 hours a week in the hospital, so we were world-weary by midway through our intern year. It is not an excuse for how we thought or talked, just some insight.

At the time Bryan was born and during his infancy, I was in my mid-30s. Bryan's mom, Olivia, was about 5 years younger than I was. I had two toddlers at the time and Olivia had three other children at home, all young. I vaguely knew that she had other children and that the family is Mormon, but I did not know much more about them even though by the middle of my second year I had cared for Bryan several times in the hospital. We all agreed that the family was nice, and my impression was that Olivia was reasonable—which was basically the highest praise a parent could get from me. Maybe still is.

Bryan, like many children with severely damaged brains, had poor overall muscle tone, upper airway obstruction, and poor airway clearance and was subject to frequent infections. Every cold became an emergency for him. He was admitted frequently to the hospital and he often ended up in the PICU because he needed more respiratory support than could be provided on the inpatient unit. When this happens, it is often difficult for parents and medical teams to admit a chronic patient like Bryan to the inpatient unit, believing that he should be sent to the PICU because "he always ends up in the PICU." This then becomes a self-fulfilling prophesy.

One night, Bryan was being admitted through the emergency department for respiratory distress. I did not feel he was sick enough to be in the PICU, so I admitted him to the inpatient unit. I was a second-year resident and was covering both the PICU and acting as the senior resident on the inpatient unit. I went to Bryan's room to explain to his mother my rationale for not admitting him to the PICU and to

© Springer Nature Switzerland AG 2021
A. F. Schrooten, B. P. Markovitz, *Shared Struggles*,
https://doi.org/10.1007/978-3-030-68020-6_13

ensure that she was comfortable with the plan. Although the hospital was fairly new and nice compared to many other hospitals, during this time we were having an odd infestation, and black flies were buzzing around several of the rooms.

I was there, in my scrubs, in the middle of the night, trying to reassure Olivia that Bryan would be monitored closely and that he would have the same medical provider (myself) in the ICU as on the inpatient unit. I arrogantly believed that I was such a superstar that Olivia should be immediately reassured by my words. At the same time, I was furiously waving away big black flies that were dive-bombing us with insect joy.

Suddenly I was struck by the absurdity. I dropped all my doctor-speak and said "I'm sure you're totally reassured with Amityville horror here. Are you buying it?" We both just started laughing. We had been holding it in with the idiot flies buzzing around and it felt great to just let it go. That moment of shared laughter was not the moment I shifted my perspective of Bryan, but it was the moment I really "saw" Olivia. We were both moms. She was a mom worried about her boy. She was doing her best to navigate the hospital and deal with yet another resident.

From that moment on, literally, we were friends. I realized that as a physician I can absolutely be professional and still be friends with the children and families I care for. While I may have known this logically, I had not felt it until that moment—the moment when through our shared laughter I saw Olivia as someone more than just a "reasonable mom." At that moment, I allowed myself to love this family, and, in doing so, I was so much more able to be myself.

Not surprisingly, Bryan ended up in the PICU that admission. Yet I did not feel as though either one of us thought that starting in the inpatient unit was the wrong thing to do. Through our initial encounter, we formed an immediate trust and understanding with each other. Despite my new found understanding, I continued to struggle with taking care of Bryan and other severely disabled children like him. I am not sure I believe in a soul in any religious way. I know there is something intangible that makes each one of us who we are, but I am quite certain that who we are lives in our brains. Without thought, without interaction with the world, and without some exchange with other humans, it is hard to be seen as "living" for me. I struggled with the time, emotional energy, and yes, money, spent in caring for Bryan when it was not clear to me that he was experiencing a life of value. In fact, I could not be sure he was not suffering through most of his life.

Olivia and Bryan's father struggled with the same questions. They absolutely believed in his soul, but they were under no delusions about his abilities. They too worried that he was unduly suffering. However, given the love they felt for him, they were unable to let him go. They struggled mightily over the decision to perform a tracheostomy and move to home ventilator support. Ultimately, they decided to move forward with aggressive intervention and support.

Over the last 2 years of my residency and into the couple of years in which I worked as a hospitalist in the PICU, I noticed a gradual shift in the way I saw Bryan. I came to see Bryan not as a child with severe disabilities but as an integral part of a large, loving family and as part of an accepting community. There was no "aha" moment; no flash of revelation. Rather, this is the nature of training. We learn physiology and pathophysiology. We learn treatment plans and diagnostic algorithms. Yet, if we are paying attention, we also learn the human component as we go along. One day we wake up and, hopefully, realize we are much better doctors—both technically and as caregivers—than we were 10 years ago or even 5 years ago. What I gained with time and experience was an appreciation of the importance of Bryan in the fabric of his family's life. He was the focus of extraordinary love and care and he helped shape the entirety of his family. They loved him simply and unconditionally.

I went on to do my fellowship in a big city near Bryan's home hospital. One night I came into the PICU for overnight call. I read ahead about the patients that were in the unit, but in the time between reading ahead and coming in for sign out, Bryan had been admitted. His home hospital PICU was full, so he was sent to our hospital. I sat down with the census list in front of me and when I saw Bryan's name, I immediately jumped up and rushed to his room.

As I entered, I did not say anything, I just went right in for a big hug with Olivia. We clung to each other, both feeling as though we felt a little bit at home in that moment. It was during that admission that Bryan had his first episodes of asystole—a long pause in his heart beating. The episodes were initially short and self-resolving but they were scary for Olivia. I was thankful that I was there to talk to her about it and prepare her for his progression.

Bryan lived several more years after that admission, bringing joy to his family. He died peacefully in his sleep when he was 9 years old. Everyone knew he had the longest, most full life he could possibly have had. In spite of her good understanding of Bryan and his limitations, the first thing Olivia said to me when we spoke was "I wasn't ready." We both knew she would never be ready.

Olivia and her husband went on to provide medical foster care and ultimately to adopt several special needs children, even as their own children were moving off to college and adulthood. We have stayed close and I have seen these new, devastated, children thrive under her care. I cannot help but be partly, secretly glad every time one of these children comes into the hospital so I can see Olivia again. There is no question that I see these children differently because of Bryan and because of Olivia.

After many years, I can see the impact that Bryan has had on my practice, most especially in the way that I view the chronically devastated children that I take care of. It remains difficult. I still remain frustrated taking care of children who live for years in chronic care facilities with little to no interaction with the world, with no family visiting or even calling. I do not think this will ever be an easy part of my job. However, I have most definitely learned to see things that early in my career I would have easily overlooked. Things such as the joy that a child brings to their family or small glimpses of the person inside that may have more awareness than is obvious at first. I have learned to listen to the parents, siblings, and loved ones and hear the story of how this child matters in their world.

Parent Commentary

I respect and appreciate this physician's honesty. She acknowledges feeling what parents of severely neurologically impaired children often sense and experience from the physicians caring for our child. It has been said that, "we don't see things as they are, we see them as we are."

Generally, physicians, especially hospital-based physicians, see our children only when they are acutely ill. They see a non-communicative, non-mobile, technology-dependent child who spends an extraordinary amount of time in the hospital taking up precious ICU bed space and resources because their fragile body is susceptible to one illness after another. In this snapshot, there is so much about our child that is not seen. Our child is not seen as having awareness; not seen as having opinions or being able to express love; and not seen as having a life of value. There is nothing more heartbreaking for a parent than to be in the care of a doctor who cannot see our child as a human being with the same feelings, emotions, and value as any other child. Physicians will question our child's quality of life without knowing anything about our child other than what is in front of them. They do not see our children in their homes, at school, or out in the community. They do not see our child's interactions with family and friends.

However, as this physician shows us, perceptions can be changed and hearts can be opened when a physician takes a moment to see their patient through the eyes of the parent. This physician took off her "doctor hat" for a brief moment and, in doing so, her perspective shifted. As she talked with Bryan's mother, mom-to-mom, she came to know Bryan as more than a severely disabled child who was sick and in the hospital all the time. She discovered how much he was cherished and valued by his parents, siblings, and community. She established a relationship with Bryan's mother that, over time, changed her perspective of Bryan and his value in this world.

The inability of a physician (or any person) to see (understand, appreciate, believe) all that we see in our children—how they communicate, display humor, and show love through their eyes, their facial expressions, and the nuances of their body language—does not negate the fact that our children *do* communicate, *do* display humor, and *do* show love. Quality of life is in the eye of the beholder. For severely disabled, medically fragile children, the parent and the child must be the ones to determine their quality of life, not the cost of care, use of resources, or an inability to understand and see our children for who they are—beautiful and cherished children whose families will go to the ends of the earth to make sure they are cared for and valued the same as any other child.

Physician Commentary

I cannot count the number of times that I have been in this physician's situation; another severely disabled, complex child with *apparently* no ability to communicate. As I hope the physicians reading this will learn—as the parents already know—just because these children do not communicate in a language that we understand, it does not mean they do not "speak a language that their families understand." Indeed, in our communications with the parents of these children, it is our profound responsibility to *understand* them—the parents—and their relationship with the child. Learn to see what they see; hear what they hear. Their senses have learned to read and communicate with their children more than we can ever do during a brief office visit or inpatient stay. At all costs, physicians need to resist the urge to state, even to themselves, *I would not do these interventions if this were my child.* Because you have never been a parent in such a situation, you cannot fathom to guess how you would behave. Do not try.

There is a more controversial aspect to this physician's story; that of becoming friends with the parent of a patient. Professional boundaries do need to be maintained for moral, ethical, and legal reasons. Friends are, by definition, biased (usually favorably) toward each other. A physician can never exhibit bias, toward or against one patient or family over another. This does not mean connections should not be created. To understand families as I describe above, a connection must be formed. I suppose it depends on a physician's definition of "friends." Forming bonds of communication and respect is healthy. Becoming true friends is risky.

Full Disclosure

14

Harlie is an amazingly resilient, adaptable, and sweet 9-year-old. She is also our medically fragile child who drew the proverbial "short straw" and was born with a multitude of birth defects. It is difficult to explain her medical complications in a way that is simple and easy to understand. The "list" of Harlie's medical complexities includes multiple heart defects, an underdeveloped right lung, spinal defects, and Goldenhar syndrome—which caused craniofacial abnormalities, including a missing ear and ear canal, an eye that does not close properly, and a severely underdeveloped jaw. Harlie has had more than 45 surgeries in her 9 years, including 5 heart surgeries, lung surgery, multiple jaw reconstruction surgeries, and spinal fusion surgery. Despite all her medical challenges, Harlie is remarkably age appropriate. She is a bright little girl with no cognitive deficits.

Because of Harlie's spinal defects, her orthopedic surgeon monitored her spine closely. When Harlie was 5 years old, the surgeon determined that surgery was necessary. The surgery involved spinal fusion and removal of vertebrae in her lumbar spine. Part of the surgery required a bone graft. When the surgeon mentioned "bone graft," I was instantly nervous.

Just a year earlier, Harlie had a second jaw reconstruction surgery that involved harvesting bone from her skull to graft onto her jaw. Harlie ended up with an infection in the bone graft. The infection traveled to her compromised heart. During surgery to clean out the infection in her jaw, Harlie went into cardiac arrest. I told the orthopedic surgeon about Harlie's history and close call. Unfortunately, we had no choice. A bone graft was the best way to achieve the best results.

Harlie had surgery at the nearest Children's Hospital equipped to handle a child with underlying cardiac issues—which was 2 hours from our home. She came out of surgery in a body cast from her armpits to her hip on one side and to her knee on the other side. She had to keep the cast on for 6 weeks. Her movement and activity were extremely limited because of the cast. It was a difficult recovery, but Harlie was in good spirits and did not complain. She was happy to lay on the couch and watch movies at home.

© Springer Nature Switzerland AG 2021
A. F. Schrooten, B. P. Markovitz, *Shared Struggles*,
https://doi.org/10.1007/978-3-030-68020-6_14

By 4 weeks post-op, Harlie was pretty itchy in the cast. She signed "itchy" and "hurt" to me. I took a long wooden q-tip and put the soft end into her cast to try and scratch her back. She cried in pain, something she rarely did. When I pulled the q-tip out it was wet with pus, and I immediately knew we were dealing with another infection. I also knew time was of the essence. I called the Children's Hospital where she had her surgery done. Because it was Saturday, I could only speak with the orthopedic resident on call. After explaining the situation, he asked me if I was a physician. I laughed and said "No." In the interest of time, he advised me to take her to the emergency department of our local hospital to be assessed.

In the emergency department, an orthopedic surgeon came to examine her. He entered the room without introducing himself to me. When I asked him who he was, he said he was the "Ortho Chief." Based on his title, I assumed he was an experienced surgeon. I explained Harlie's history and my concerns. He was confident that it was just a minor irritation and it was nothing to be concerned about. He told me:

Fluid follows gravity. If it were serious, we would see fluid gathering at the bottom of her incision.

Her incision was more than 6 inches long and we could only see the bottom tip of it. What about the rest of the incision?

She would have a fever.

I explained that she had a major infection in her jaw 9 weeks post-op after bone graft jaw reconstruction surgery last year, and when the surgeon did an irrigation and debridement, she coded and went into cardiac arrest. Never once did she have a fever. In fact, she has not had a fever—at all—in over 2 years.

She would be less active and/or lethargic.

She was in a body cast and could not move, whether she had energy or not. She was also a kid with major heart and lung defects and she never had a lot of energy because of them. In my opinion, this was not something that could rule out the possibility of something serious brewing.

She would have a loss in appetite.

She has a G-tube and has been tube fed all of her life. We only recently got her to a point where she would take some of her nutrition orally, in pureed form. Again, this was not a relevant indicator in Harlie's case.

After our discussions, the doctor called the orthopedic resident on call at the Children's Hospital to discuss the matter. He returned to our exam room to tell us they were in agreement and we should go home and be seen in the clinic by her surgeon on Wednesday—which was 4 days away. I was not happy with this plan. Based on our past experience with a very similar situation, I felt it was too risky. I asked about cutting the cast to get a better look at the incision. He told me he did not think that was necessary. He was extremely confident this was not something to be overly concerned about. At that point, I knew this doctor and this hospital could not help us. I also knew this was no minor skin irritation.

The following Monday morning, I made the 2 hour drive to take Harlie to the emergency department at Children's Hospital. Waiting until Wednesday for an appointment with her surgeon was not an option. Someone needed to cut the cast and see the surgical site as soon as possible.

Harlie's surgeon came to see us in the emergency department. She was not easily convinced. After all, Harlie had no visible symptoms. I stated my case, confident that something was wrong. She trusted my knowledge of Harlie and my gut feeling that something was wrong and agreed to cut the cast. At the very top of her incision there was an area of necrotic tissue larger than the size of a quarter—it looked like a hole. Harlie's surgeon was visibly shocked. It was a very serious infection and meant Harlie had to have surgery that night. By the time the surgical team was prepped and ready to go, it was after nine o'clock.

Knowing that Harlie went into cardiac arrest the last time this happened, I was terrified. I was so afraid we were going to lose her that night. I cried as I told her I loved her, said goodbye, and handed her over to the operating team. All the doctors involved in her case were very compassionate and made sure I knew she was in good hands. They took every precaution possible knowing her history.

I waited anxiously. After 4 hours, surgery was finished and Harlie was okay. Her surgeon reopened the incision completely, cleaned the wound, and removed the dead bone graft. She put in a wound VAC, packed the wound with a spongelike material, and connected the wound VAC to suction equipment. Over the next 9 days, Harlie went back to the operating room to repeat the debridement process four more times! It was a grueling recovery, even for a little girl who had been through more than her fair share of surgeries and difficult recoveries. Harlie's surgeon said that if we had waited any longer, the outcome could have been catastrophic.

One of my biggest regrets following this event was not contacting the doctor who saw Harlie in the emergency department of our local hospital. He did not "hear" me and was dangerously over confident. Even though he introduced himself as the "Ortho Chief," I found out later that he should have said Ortho Chief *Resident*. To an experienced parent like myself, that is an important distinction. He misrepresented himself, not just to me, but also to the resident at our Children's Hospital. I believe had the resident at Children's known he was speaking to someone with comparable experience he would have sought advice from a more experienced attending physician. Had I been less knowledgeable or less confident and done what he advised, Harlie may not have survived.

Parent Commentary

Parents of medically complex children can spend weeks and months at a time living in the hospital with their child, oftentimes beginning with the birth of their child and continuing throughout their child's life. One of the first things we learn is medical hierarchy. We quickly learn the titles "resident," "fellow," and "attending," and over time we learn the knowledge and experience that comes with each one of those titles. We also become the experts when it comes to our own child, and our knowledge and experience should be respected, especially when dealing with an acute or out-of-the-norm-for-our-child issue.

Because we spend so much time in and out of hospitals and interacting with doctors, we take our child to the emergency department as a last resort and only after we have done everything in our power to manage the issue on our own—for the very reason that our concerns are often discounted by those who do not know us or our child. When we seek help with an acute issue, we have a true understanding that the issue we are concerned about is serious.

In this story, you have a child with significant medical complexity and a very knowledgeable mother. I believe it is appropriate and necessary for the orthopedic resident to disclose his accurate title. Providing this information to the parent does not diminish the role of the resident, rather it gives the parent information needed to ask the appropriate questions and make informed decisions based on the information provided. Some issues need the knowledge of a more experienced physician and the parent has the right to know the level of experience of the physician they are dealing with. Had Harlie's mother known she was dealing with a resident, she likely would have asked to see the orthopedic attending on call.

While I believe the orthopedic resident should have disclosed his accurate title to Harlie's mother, the bigger issue is that he did not appreciate that Harlie's mother was the expert when it came to her child. She conveyed enough information to the resident about Harlie's prior life-threatening experience involving a bone graft that it should have caught his attention that she knew what she was talking about. Acknowledging that parents are the experts of their medically complex child is a skill that comes with time and experience in caring for this unique population of patients and their parents. This physician was not there yet and it could have cost Harlie her life. If parents are to trust doctors, then doctors—especially less experienced doctors—need to trust parents.

Physician Commentary

This is a painful story to read. I cannot count the number of times an overconfident junior physician discounted the appropriate concerns of a highly knowledgeable parent. We are taught in medical school: listen to the patient. They know themselves the best. In pediatrics, the parent is usually the proxy for their child and especially in medically complex children, parents are—in my experience—almost always right. They are at least correct in their concerns that something serious is wrong, even if they may not know what exactly is the nature of the problem. Figuring out the problem, based on the parent concern, is the job of the doctor!

There is also an element to this story that may be at play. We do not truly know the training level or, more importantly, the pediatric experience of the "ortho chief" at the local hospital. Surgeons who specialize in pediatric care, of course, spend tremendous amount of time training with children, but a surgeon at a community hospital may have had only a relatively brief time training in the pediatric domain. Having said this, an orthopedic residency training program is at least 5 years long after medical school, and this physician, as a "chief," was likely at least in year 5 if not engaged in an extra year beyond that. (I am not an orthopedic surgeon and do not play one on TV so do not quote me on this!)

In my experience in pediatric academic medicine, pediatricians and pediatric specialists are getting better over time in trusting the instincts of parents of medically complex children. Frankly, I am not sure this trend applies quite as well to surgeons. We have an inside joke in pediatrics about surgeons: sometimes wrong, never in doubt. Of course I am over-generalizing, but hearing this story only confirms this bias for me.

With respect to knowing the medical hierarchy, e.g., resident, fellow, and attending, many institutions now require all physicians and staff to wear a badge that extends below their personal name badge that states their role. Mine says "attending doctor" and the pediatric critical care fellow with me today has one that states "fellow doctor." We like to think this overtly lets patients and families know our roles, but this also assumes they know the differences.

Finally, every parent of a medically complex child must have a strong ally "on the inside" (of the medical system) and no doubt most do, e.g., their pediatrician, their neurologist, and their pulmonologist. In situations like this when they are hitting a brick wall, my advice would be to "phone a friend" and get your "inside partner" to help advocate with you and for your child.

The Photograph

15

It was a photograph that made me shudder. It was a photograph that made me question. It was a photograph that made me smile.

Early in my critical care fellowship, I received a premature infant from a local NICU for planned surgical procedures—a gastrostomy placement and inguinal hernia reduction. Tommy had significant bronchopulmonary dysplasia, feeding intolerance, and the other "routine" issues that one might expect for his gestational age. While I do not recall all the details of the postoperative course, it was not without complications. There were definitely challenges obtaining vascular access. His pulmonary mechanics and gas exchange were worse than expected, or at least than I expected. Sedation was a nightmare. At this time, we were still using food coloring dye to assess feeding tolerance, reflux, and aspiration. Tommy's mom will never let me forget that someone (me?) stained his favorite stuffed animal—a hungry caterpillar—with blue dye on the nose. It took several weeks for Tommy to settle down, but he eventually returned to his home NICU.

That winter, however, I met my little friend again. This was not an elective admission. It was dire. RSV had derailed his convalescence. The transport team called in advance about possible ECMO. I stood at bed space 12a (there was no bed space 13) with one of our respiratory therapists as he taught me about lung hyperinflation, cardiopulmonary interactions, and that "less may be more" when it comes to ventilator support. This admission was again a protracted course for Tommy, but "my" little guy made a slow recovery. With his parents by his side, Tommy eventually transitioned to a local rehabilitation facility for long-term ventilator weaning and preparation for home care.

As my second year of fellowship began, I took advantage of an opportunity to run an inpatient rehabilitation unit. Alternating between the ICU and rehab provided me with continuity and the possibility for assessing long-term outcomes, combining my interest in acute and chronic care. Who was there to greet me on my first day, but my former preemie friend, Tommy, and his parents. In fact, he was my first "project."

© Springer Nature Switzerland AG 2021   73
A. F. Schrooten, B. P. Markovitz, *Shared Struggles*,
https://doi.org/10.1007/978-3-030-68020-6_15

I joined an amazing team and watched as Tommy literally grew into readiness for home. During this time, Tommy's mom experienced some of her own medical issues, which were likely compounded by fatigue from balancing work and time at Tommy's bedside in rehab. I went to visit her when she was hospitalized. She was threatening to leave to see her son and needed reassurance that he was okay and, yet, she needed to focus on getting herself better. It was my first insight into how much of a toll prematurity and the resulting chronic conditions had taken on the family.

After several months in the rehabilitation unit, Tommy was stable enough to go home. A few weeks after his discharge, I received a thank-you note with a picture inside. There they were, mom and Tommy in the backyard pool. Tommy was in a float ring and respiratory tubing could be seen extending to the edge of the pool and beyond the frame of the photo.

My first reaction was a sinking feeling. This was not safe. Are they crazy? Do I call child protective services? Why would they do this, the pool and the picture? Despite my initial thoughts, as I continued to stare at the picture I could not help but smile. The other thought that came to me was, "He looks good!" His mom's smile was huge. I could only imagine how happy his dad, a techie, was to be using his fancy camera for the special occasion.

Throughout my years of practice, I have received many pictures of my long-term, chronic patients. Pictures of kids with ventilators on rollercoasters, on top of mountains, canoeing, and simply being with their families. They are just doing what kids do. What I have learned is that technology is a means to an end, and that end is being together as a family and living life to the fullest.

It was a photograph that helped me understand. It remains a photograph that motivates me to this day.

Parent Commentary

When our children are discharged from the hospital connected to ICU-level equipment and needing ICU-level care, we cannot begin to imagine how we will ever be able to participate in life as we knew it before we became a "medical family." Suctioning machines, ventilators, feeding pumps, and central lines do not create a picture of mobility, joy, or normalcy.

There is a definite learning curve during those first months home as we focus on learning the equipment and keeping our child alive. We take baby steps. We feel a sense of accomplishment just moving our child from room to room in our home. Then we master loading the ventilator, suction machine, feeding pump, medical supply bag, back-up equipment bag, and normal baby stuff bag on the stroller and somehow find room for the baby in there to brave a walk in the neighborhood. Eventually, we risk venturing beyond the comfort of our home base to participate in family and community activities. We ease into our new normal and find a way to participate in life again.

It is not surprising that Tommy's doctor was alarmed when he saw a picture of a ventilator-dependent child in a swimming pool. It was probably not something Tommy's parents even thought possible during those early days in the rehab hospital. I would guess that the ultimate goal of the physician is to get the child stable enough to leave the hospital and be at home with their family. However, what the reality of being at home encompasses is probably not given much thought. The ultimate goal of the parents is to find joy in life despite the challenges of their new normal. It is important for parents to share what life outside of the hospital looks like for their child. Pictures of our child participating in activities and enjoying life are not only encouraging for other parents who are just beginning this journey, they also let the doctors know that helping us to get our child home—even with all the technology required—is a gift, and we are grateful for everything they do to make it a reality. Additionally, as Tommy's doctor tells us, when we share images and stories of our joy-filled life outside of the confines of the hospital, it encourages doctors because they can see that their efforts matter and make a positive difference in the lives of their patients and their patient's families. Parents of medically complex children are resilient and creative and, with technology and the care and support of our child's doctors, the possibilities are endless as we strive to give our child the best possible life.

Physician Commentary

What life is like for families and children with complex medical conditions is often a blind spot for pediatric and neonatal intensive care physicians. Yes, we work hard with our families and talented multidisciplinary teams to get these children home, but most of us have little idea what happens after we wave goodbye from the ICU. This physician, perhaps due to his ability to also spend time with such children in rehabilitation, has developed a stronger line of sight on what "home" really means. Too often, our next contact with these children is when they need readmission to the ICU for a complication or an intercurrent illness. So we continue to put them into our "sick child" paradigm.

My hope is that more communication from such children and their families to their ICU physicians will occur. It is incredibly important for ICU physicians and the entire ICU team to receive these pictures and stories. It brightens our days and gives fresh meaning to the work we do. It opens our eyes to a new paradigm: that our most complex and technology-dependent children can still be children, living life to the fullest extent and bringing joy to their loved ones.

Learning Together

16

"It's kind of like backpacking in Europe, isn't it?" chuckled a woman with frazzled hair (much like my own), brushing her teeth in the Children's Hospital bathroom. I let out a laugh for the first time in what felt like months. Yes, that was an appropriate comparison. Literally *living* in the hospital with your medically fragile child was a lot like living out of a backpack for an extended stay in a foreign land. Except for all of the obvious fun stuff—you trade the Louvre for the lab and the Mona Lisa for monitors. The only souvenirs you return home with are in the form of scars, both emotional and physical.

Our daughter Addison was born at 24 weeks gestation following a tumultuous pregnancy riddled with complications that lead to her premature birth. She spent the first 6 months of her life in the Neonatal Intensive Care Unit (NICU) where she underwent a PDA ligation, two laser eye surgeries to ease her Stage 3 ROP (retinopathy of prematurity) with Plus Disease and a G-tube placement. After many failed attempts at having the breathing tube removed, she received a tracheostomy when she was 6 months old. Shortly after getting the trach, Addison was discharged from the NICU only to land in the emergency department of a more specialized Children's Hospital 24 later. We spent an additional 8 months at Children's Hospital until Addison stabilized enough to come home.

It was interactions like I had with the fellow parent in the bathroom that one morning that made residing in the hospital the first 14 months of Addison's life bearable. If we were lucky, we would have chance encounters with others who "got it." Because we were mostly sequestered to our rooms, whether it be because our child was on contact precautions or tethered to a ventilator, we had limited interactions with the outside world. Most of the other families who found themselves on our floor were there for temporary stays as the rooms around us were filled and emptied within 24 hours. Certain signs signaled that a family was in store for a long-term stay—a decorated door, the medical team on a first name basis with a family. Then there was the sign that felt like a boulder was lodged in the pit of your stomach—a room filled with extended family hovering over a child in their bed. Breaking the hospital's limit of two visitors per patient could only mean the unthinkable—a

© Springer Nature Switzerland AG 2021   77
A. F. Schrooten, B. P. Markovitz, *Shared Struggles*,
https://doi.org/10.1007/978-3-030-68020-6_16

family was going to be leaving the hospital without their child. A few months after our encounter in the bathroom, I stopped seeing the mom with whom I shared the brief light moment about traveling and learned she had tragically lost her daughter. This was not Europe, it was hell.

Needless to say, living life in a hospital can be rather depressing. Often times, doctors rounding in the morning were your first sign of interaction with the outside world. Even though you knew your "sentence," the brief encounter with the medical team was like going before the parole board. Jailbreak was always the goal, but rarely ever the outcome of the day. Being at a teaching hospital, the medical team rotated every 4–6 weeks. It did not take long to establish favorite attending physicians. Then there were the residents. What they lacked in experience they often overcompensated for in confidence. Unlike the attendings who would cycle back on to the floor, residents would only spend a week at a time on your floor. Telling a new fresh-faced resident your child's whole history at the start of each week's rotation knowing that you would never see them beyond the week became exhausting. Having them challenge your thoughts and opinions was maddening. We felt like our daughter was a subject in a classroom and the residents were the dreaded substitutes.

During Addison's long admission at Children's, we learned that her breathing issues were more complex than just needing a stable airway. Her lung disease, made more severe from months on the oscillating ventilator, needed long-term mechanical ventilation. Thus, we added a home ventilator to our arsenal of medical supplies. When it was finally time for discharge, we were not thrilled that we were assigned to a newly graduated fellow, which was a slight step above a resident in our opinion. The other attending physicians' caseloads were full, and this newly appointed pulmonologist needed patients.

Prior to being assigned to Dr. B, our experience with him was limited. When we showed up for our first post-discharge office visit, he seemed nervous and quiet. We did take notice of the way he interacted with Addison. Although she was mostly noninteractive at that point, he attempted to play peek-a-boo with her and, well, treated her like a baby. The next year was full of repeat hospital admissions for respiratory issues related to Addison's chronic lung disease. With every single one of these admissions, whether it be for 24 hours or 24 days, Dr. B stopped by our room. He was not always on service, but he made it a part of his day to come see Addison. He would talk with us about nonmedical things, whether it commenting on a basketball game that was on TV or a book that one of us was reading while Addison slept.

When it came time to make decisions in the next steps in Addison's care, such as weaning the ventilator or oxygen, he always asked us what our thoughts were. Sometimes this was irritating. Were we not seeing him so he could tell us what the next steps were? Later we appreciated his confidence in our decision-making, as we were able to wean Addison off the ventilator quicker than most doctors would have wanted. When it came time for her to be off the ventilator for longer periods of time, we mentioned to him that we needed an order for a medical humidifier for her trach because she was no longer going to be receiving humidity from the heater on the ventilator. Dr. B seemed more confident than usual and told us a humidifier was not needed. While my husband and I are not doctors, we received our education from personal experience and from an online network of other parents whose children had trachs. We knew Addison needed the humidifier. When we brought this to his attention, Dr. B quickly dismissed himself. Twenty minutes later, he returned and offered an apology. We were correct, Addison did need a humidifier. What struck me the most about this interaction was not that he did not know the equipment Addison needed, but that when he had a question, he sought the answer and was not too prideful to admit he was wrong.

As the years went by, Addison was weaned off the ventilator and her trach was removed. Our visits to see Dr. B in the pulmonary department decreased, but he still stayed in touch with us. When Addison underwent a routine bronch, before he gave us the results, he expressed his condolences for a recent pregnancy loss we experienced. He heard the news through a nurse who has stayed in contact with us. He did not shy away from an opportunity to connect. He saw us as people first, a patient second.

A few years ago when Addison underwent a procedure to have a permanent cecostomy tube placed, we never heard from or saw the GI doctor after the surgery and weeklong hospital stay. When we arrived home and the hospital's familiar number appeared on my phone, I was expecting it to be the GI department. Nope, it was Dr. B's nurse. He had been out of town, heard about Addison's procedure and wanted to see how she was recovering. This was not his department or responsibility to check on her, but that is what he did because that is just what he does.

Although Dr. B was seeking new patients when he was out fresh out of his fellowship, an appointment with him now requires a 6-month wait. An appointment with him also often requires a long wait in the waiting room as he is always running behind. More relaxed and settled into my role as a mom of a medically fragile child, I now smile as we wait and picture other families getting the same level of personal care we have received over the years. Perhaps he is on the floor seeing a patient or just taking his time to answer someone's questions in the next room. Some doctors are worth waiting for.

What has always stood out about Dr. B is his humanness. Is he the most knowledgeable pulmonary doctor on staff? Probably not. The most experienced? Not even close. Neither is he some idyllic Patch Adams, but he connects with his patients and their families. When Addison was first discharged from Children's as a baby and we were assigned to the least experienced pulmonologist in the group, we—Addison's parents and her doctor—were all rookies at caring for a medically fragile and complex child. We listened to each other, we learned together, and we came to trust each other. Dr. B understands and acknowledges that our lived experience in managing Addison's medical needs over the years carries equal weight with what was learned in medical school. Dr. B's willingness to be vulnerable, to admit when he is wrong, and his taking time to know us, not just as parents of a patient, but as people with common interests, displays a rare humanity that is often missing in the doctor-patient relationship. This humanity stands out. This humanity is instrumental in creating a trusting relationship, and a trusting relationship with your child's doctor is essential when you have a child with a chronic complex condition that will require a lifetime of medical care.

Living a life filled with hospital stays and doctors' appointments is certainly a far cry from the excitement of backpacking through a foreign land. However, we have been fortunate to have crossed paths with Dr. B—a very special doctor who has lightened the load on our journey and made each step on the path a little easier.

Parent Commentary

Parents of medically complex children spend an extraordinary amount of time interacting with their child's team of doctors. This team can include as many as ten or more specialists. When you spend so much time seeing the same doctors over the course of many years—the connection with these doctors is very special, almost sacred. It is not realistic to expect to have the kind of relationship that Addison's parents had with Dr. B with every doctor on our child's care team, but when we do find that one special doctor we can connect with, it makes all the difference in the world to us.

Our children are more than a list of anomalies and conditions, we are more than the parent of a sick child, and our child's doctor is more than just a provider of information and treatments. We are human beings first. Addison's parents connected with Dr. B because he recognized this. He took the time to get to know a little about them and he allowed them to get to know a little about him. As a young and inexperienced doctor, he welcomed their knowledge and input and he did not pretend to be the expert. The rare doctor who (figuratively) takes off his or her white coat and connects with the parent as one vulnerable human to another creates a trust that is instrumental to the parents over the course of their child's life.

There will be times when we will question or disagree with our child's doctors and times when we are not certain what the next step in their care should be. When we have that one doctor we can trust, the one doctor who can be our go-to and who will be honest, yet compassionate, we are much more likely to listen to what they have to say and respect their opinion, even if we disagree with it or it is something we do not want to hear. Trust is one of the most important factors in the relationship with our child's doctor. If a parent has to choose between the doctor we trust and the doctor who is more experienced or skilled, we will almost always choose the doctor we trust. Of course, the best case scenario is when the doctor we trust is also the doctor with the most experience. Although, as Addison's story shows us, if you are fortunate, you find that doctor you trust, you stick together and, eventually, he or she will inevitably become the doctor with the most experience.

Physician Commentary

Physicians learn as much from their patients and patients' families, if not more so, than from their training. Medical school and postgraduate training is really nothing more than a driver's license. Yes, you can "practice" medicine legally, but I have joked over the years that I am still "practicing," in the sense that I have still not gotten it right. Furthermore, there is a famous parable in medicine that the Dean of Harvard Medical School once told the graduating class (paraphrased): "Half of what we taught you these last four years will be proven false. The bad news is, we don't know which half."

The comment that struck me deeply from this story, was about residents. "Then there were the residents. What they lacked in experience they often overcompensated for in confidence." Doctors are taught that they are the "experts" and need to have the answers. Well—"light bulb" (thank you Dr. Gru in "Despicable Me")—this just is not so. The field of medicine is advancing so rapidly, exponentially even, that no one physician can have a glimmer of hope to keep up alone. They need partners. And in the world of medically complex and fragile children, I am sure by now the reader can guess who those partners are. There is no human on earth more invested in the care of a child than that child's parent. And with the world of information (admittedly, some valid and some bogus) available now to anyone with an Internet connection, physicians can and must rely on parents as partners in the journey of these children.

Finally, humility is a rare but vital characteristic for physicians caring for such children. Humility says: "I do not have the answer, let's find it together." As you can see from this story and others, humility in a physician is decidedly not a sign of weakness, but rather the bravest sign of strength.

Altered Path

17

I am a pediatric pulmonologist. I became a pediatrician because I love working with children and, I will admit, because I have much less patience with adults. In my early years of practice, my interests and expertise were children with cystic fibrosis, chronic lung disease of premature infants, and critically ill children on home ventilators.

Then I met Emma.

I was running the Pediatric Intensive Care Unit in a private hospital and building my pediatric pulmonary practice when Emma was admitted to the hospital with pneumonia. Emma was 2 years old—a tiny, blond-haired, fair-skinned little girl with a big personality. She was born with spinal muscular atrophy (SMA) Type 2, an inherited disease that causes progressive muscle weakness.

Emma was discharged from the hospital after a few days. However, once home, her mother, Sally, was concerned because she was still struggling with increased work of breathing, difficulty clearing her secretions, and a cough. Worried about what she should do, Sally called another mother of a child with SMA and asked for advice. She told Sally to take Emma back to the hospital's emergency department, ask for me and do not leave until Emma was seen by me. It worked. I saw Emma that day in the emergency department and so began my adventure into the world of Sally and Emma, SMA, and neuromuscular disease.

Emma recovered from her bout of pneumonia, but more episodes were to follow. Her mother began researching on her own and attended a meeting for families of children with SMA. One of the speakers was a physician who dealt with muscle weakness in many forms. He was an expert in noninvasive ventilation and secretion clearance. At the meeting, he mentioned a cough assist device called an *insufflator-exsufflator*. The device simulates a deep cough by using pressure. It was created originally to help polio patients, but had fallen out of use with the development of the polio vaccine and decline of polio cases. Sally came to me and asked if this equipment would help Emma.

© Springer Nature Switzerland AG 2021
A. F. Schrooten, B. P. Markovitz, *Shared Struggles*,
https://doi.org/10.1007/978-3-030-68020-6_17

Sally is a strong and determined mother who would do anything and everything to help Emma. When she approached me about the cough assist device, I was apprehensive. I was afraid that I would disappoint her if I was not able to get the information she needed, or if the device would not benefit Emma or, even worse, if it harmed her. However, I listened because this was a mother fighting for her child's quality of life with all she had. Sally was Emma's strongest advocate and, as Emma's physician, I knew it was important to listen, keep an open mind, and support her.

I had never heard of the cough assist machine, but immediately began to research it. The equipment company was very helpful and provided me with two machines, one for me to use for practice and one to use for teaching. I also read articles written by the physician who had significant experience with the equipment and its use on patients with neuromuscular weakness. I went to one of his lectures, bought his book, and even called him. The patience of this family and their trust drove me to learn more. Sally and I learned to use the cough assist together. With perseverance, we fine-tuned the settings and finally started seeing a difference in Emma's overall health.

By word of mouth, particularly Emma's and Sally's, interest in the cough assist spread throughout the muscular dystrophy population locally. I started to see more patients with muscle weakness from muscular dystrophies, SMA, myopathies, cerebral palsy, and spinal cord injuries. I became active in the Muscular Dystrophy Association (MDA) camp and MDA fundraising. I left private practice and joined the faculty at the Children's Hospital. I became an expert on respiratory complications and treatments in children with neuromuscular diseases. I started a clinic for children who were technology dependent. Beyond the opportunity to help these families, the most gratifying was to be chosen as a member of a standards of care committee that gave me the incredible experience of meeting international leaders of all aspects of muscle disease.

Emma and Sally changed the direction of my career and taught me so much along the way. When asked to pursue the use of a device I had not heard of and had no experience with, it would have been easier to take the "I do not have time for this" path and stick with what I knew and had experience with. Yet, listening to Sally and honoring her commitment to provide Emma with the best quality of life possible was one of the best investments of my time I have ever made. I am thankful to them for being a part of my career and life's journey.

I recently visited Emma in her apartment near the university she attends while getting her graduate degree in public administration. She plans to use her education to help others who have similar challenges. She lives with a roommate and has caretakers that help her throughout the day and night. I was thrilled when she showed me she had the most recent version of the cough assist machine which she uses faithfully to keep her lungs healthy.

Parent Commentary

One of the first things that parents of children with rare diseases do is find each other. We look to each other for support and information. Together we find the best doctors for our child's disease, whether it be locally or across the country. We endlessly research, find, and read about the most current and proven treatments and interventions. The parent in this story reached out to another parent and was directed to ask to be seen by a specific physician and to not leave the hospital until her child was seen by that physician. Whether it was luck that this physician was in the hospital and available the day Emma's mother took her to the emergency department, or whether a message was conveyed to the physician that another patient's mother recommended her and this physician honored the referral, it was, nevertheless, a transformative encounter for both patient and physician.

When your child has a rare and life-limiting condition, it is not only important to find other families who are traveling the same path, it is equally as important to find a physician who will walk alongside you and your child through it all—the sick days, the stable days, the successes, and the challenges. Parents are their child's fiercest advocate, but parents also need a physician on their team who will advocate for their child. When new treatments and technologies become available, physicians hold the key to a patient's access to those treatments and technologies. Making that one connection with the right physician can be life changing for the patient and the patient's family and, as this story shows us, it can also be life changing for the physician.

This story is not only about a patient who changed the course of a physician's career, it is a story of a physician who trusted a parent's knowledge and was willing to risk going from what she knew and currently practiced to take the time to learn something new and outside of her established area of practice. The physician in this story exemplifies the physician advocate that all children with a chronic complex medical condition needs on their team.

Physician Commentary

This story is inspiring as a physician because this is the kind of doctor all doctors want to be; one who listens to patients and families, trusts that the parents know their child the best, and recognizes their own limitations and blind spots.

What a physician learns in medical school and in their training only takes them so far. Medical advances, or in this case, rediscovery of older "innovations," continue to expand rapidly. Physicians truly must be life-long learners, but this story reminds us it is not just textbooks and medical journals that we must learn from. We must partner with our patients and families to keep learning, keeping our minds open.

A physician might see 20 patients in a day, but to a parent of a chronically ill child, they only see one "patient" and they see that "patient" day and night. Especially in our interconnected world, parents have the resources to research their child's condition and network with other families. They need their physicians to listen to them and help them evaluate the information they have discovered. And as this story shows us, that evaluation should happen as partners.

The Befores and the Afters

18

The Joint Commission, the organization that accredits and certifies health care orga-
nizations in the United States, defines a sentinel event as "an unexpected occurrence
involving death or serious physical or psychological injury." As a pediatric epilepsy
specialist who spends the bulk of my time in the Pediatric and Neonatal Intensive
Care Units, I am the physical embodiment of a sentinel event. I am frequently a part
of an experience that clearly divides a family's life into a "before" and an "after"
and permanently alters the reality they have known.

I met Will as a frail, intubated 5-day old, his red hair a vivid contrast against his
crisp white sheet. The Neonatal Intensive Care Unit (NICU) requested my consultation because he had a rare genetic mutation and was having very long, frequent
seizures. The high doses of seizure medications Will received prior to transfer were
sedating, and he rested in the warmth of his incubator, unmoving. His mother held
vigil by his bed, drained of color except for her bloodshot eyes and the matching
hair she shared with her son.

Although unexpectedly thrust into the harsh reality of the NICU, Will's mother
adapted. The background rhythm of his ventilator punctuated our lengthy daily visits as we painstakingly reviewed Will's past 24 hours and discussed the changes in
his care plan. Initially, desperation and distrust drove her to tireless online research.
Will's birth hospital had not been receptive to her assertions that something was
wrong. Empowered by family-centered rounds, her motivation slowly changed.
Now she was driven to become an expert in her son, studying each new medication
and learning how to optimize his specialized ketogenic diet. She gradually built the
knowledge base that would allow her to manage his seizures with us on the phone,
instead of at his bedside.

With time, Will's mother started to share her other stresses with me: how her
other kids were confused by the fact that she was too scared to leave Will's side and
go home. How her husband was struggling to hold their life outside the hospital
together. How hard it was even for her parents, Will's grandparents, to understand
what his little body was going through, what she as a mother was going through, and
why we, as his doctors, could not stop his seizures.

© Springer Nature Switzerland AG 2021   87
A. F. Schrooten, B. P. Markovitz, *Shared Struggles*,
https://doi.org/10.1007/978-3-030-68020-6_18

I was rounding on Will at the exact moment of the Boston Marathon bombing. She watched my face with concern as I paused, distracted by the alert ribbon scrolling across the small TV screen in Will's room. She intuitively asked, "How many people do you know that are running today?" My sisters, my husband, and I have all been runners since high school, and my heart raced as I grasped for the list of friends who had qualified for Boston that year. Flustered, I answered a shaky, "I really don't know." The following day, the second I entered Will's room, his mother inquired if my family and friends were okay. We had truly become a health care team. We cared about Will, and we cared about each other.

Will's discharge day finally arrived. His mother, armed with seizure rescue medications and our cell phone numbers, was thrilled to be taking her 5-month-old son home. The nurses were evenly divided; half hoped for the best, half cynically predicted immediate re-admission. In the 3 months that Will was at home with his family, his mother became an expert at managing Will's daily seizures. A few times each week she called the neurologist on call for support during Will's prolonged nighttime events. While she gave Will the additional medications we advised and we waited together on the phone for his seizures to stop, she would share the challenges of taking her medically complex baby to his sister's soccer games and ask how her favorite nurses were doing. Our outpatient clinic visits opened with a round of hugs from the team and a group viewing of the latest and cutest cell phone pictures of Will and his siblings.

One winter evening, Will's mother called as she was speeding back to the emergency room. Will was having trouble breathing. I rolled out of bed, pulled on the first clothes I could reach and was shivering while racing down an empty interstate when the PICU resident paged me. As I entered the familiar unit, the nurses knowingly nodded me toward his room. Initially, we sat in Will's room as doctor, mother, and patient. However, when night descends on a hospital, the lights dim, the pace calms, and the conversations grow quieter and more intimate. We became two people—two mothers—sitting by the bed of a baby with an unspoken understanding that this would be the last time. She reminisced about his pregnancy and delivery and we stroked his wispy auburn curls. Night yielded to a peaceful dawn and she shared that she could feel Will growing tired. Her heart was heavy with the knowledge that Will was ready to stop fighting. During a tearful hug, she asked me to let the PICU team know that it was time to extubate and we each said our quiet goodbyes.

Will lives on in our hospital. He is in the memories of snuggles with nurses while his mom refreshed her coffee, in the care package program his mom started on our epilepsy unit, and in the residents' composure during a patient's long seizures. These things are Will's legacy. We are carrying forward his "after."

As a part of a medical team, even as I do my best to support families, I cannot fully understand what it means to have a child go through an illness or an injury that takes their life. I cannot understand what it means to say goodbye to your child and have that part of you that exists outside your body leave. I will forever be in awe of Will's mother's strength and grace and how she changed, always evolving to become the parent he needed. Every time, including the final time, she chose Will's needs over her own.

Walking this journey with Will's family, and other families, has helped me understand how to love fiercely and how to gracefully let go; how to honor the children we love and affectionately remember the children we have lost. These experiences have made me truly grateful for the privilege of being a part of the "befores" and the "afters." I still struggle with the fact that the day I meet many families is a day that forever changes their lives. I hope they can take solace, as I do, in the knowledge that caring for their children forever changes my life too.

Parent Commentary

This story shares the important message that even though doctors in certain specialties have to routinely deliver devastating news to parents about their child's condition, the fact that it is routine does not make it easy; it does not mean doctors are not affected by the impact of the diagnoses they deliver to their patient's families. However, I also believe that many of us who have received a life-altering and/or life-limiting diagnosis for our child do not see the impact on the doctor delivering the devastating news because they generally do not reveal to us what they are feeling. Sometimes the lack of emotion by the doctor can unfairly be translated by a parent to mean that the doctor has no empathy or compassion. Yet, I can understand the need for doctors to protect their own mental health by keeping some distance and not allowing themselves to be emotionally attached to every patient and family they have to deliver a life-changing diagnosis to. This story, however, shares the rewards of opening your heart and being a part of the "after."

The doctor in this story recognizes that, because of the nature of her specialty, she is often the messenger of bad news that changes families' lives forever. Yet, she does not close her heart to the suffering of her patients and their parents despite the fact that their pain is something she routinely witnesses. Doctors can be more than bearers of information; they have the opportunity to be an important part of what happens after they deliver a diagnosis if they are willing to risk giving of their time and their heart. This doctor gave both to Will's mother and, as a result, a trusting relationship and unique doctor-parent bond was established. This bond allowed Will's mother to freely and comfortably share the struggles and challenges of life outside of the hospital. In turn, by allowing herself to be part of Will's "after" and forming a bond with his mother, this doctor was touched and changed by their story.

We all want to believe that our child came into this world to make a difference—it is how we find purpose and meaning in our "after." We know our child makes a profound difference in our life. But when we hear that our child's life also makes a meaningful and lasting impact on the lives of the doctors who care for them, it touches our heart and makes our child's fragile and, all too often, short life all the more cherished.

Physician Commentary

It should not surprise us when two human beings connect at a, well, human level. When life deals us a stressful blow, it is a basic instinct to seek connections with others who can understand and empathize. What could be more stressful than a life-altering diagnosis for your child? Who could best understand the implications of this diagnosis than your child's physician? Still, it remains mysterious to me the precise combination of circumstances (and stars?) that must align for the type of connection described in this story to occur. I would hope that of the multiple physicians that parents of children with complex medical conditions encounter, they are able to form this kind of bond with at least one along the way. I wish I could offer a prescription for how to make this happen. To this day, I remain befuddled how I made a connection to the mom of a little boy named Jack, and this book is a consequence of that connection.

In any case, every interaction of a physician with a family, especially those with these complicated and fragile patients, can and should be one of compassion and empathy. Although in this case a connection beyond the medical care of the patient was made, this level of communication is not necessary to offer heartfelt support and appreciation of the magnitude of the impact of the child's illness on the family. I have said it before and will say it again here, patients and families do not care how much you know until they know how much you care.

Not Everyone Is Born a Superhero

19

I was at home, the night before my shift in the Pediatric Intensive Care Unit. As a more junior attending physician, I like to prepare myself the day before any clinical work by reading through the active patient census. This gives me the time to digest the complexity of the care I will undoubtedly have to provide to all my patients. As I scrolled through the list, a name jumped out at me. Almost 5 months prior, Yessica—a spunky adolescent, was admitted to my ICU with a new diagnosis of a brain aneurysm and stroke. Quirky with a grim sense of humor, upon meeting me for the very first time she cautiously asked, "Do patients die in this room?" I chuckled and told her, "Of course not! Patients come here to get better." She did remarkably well at the time, but carried a much higher lifetime risk of complications down the road.

Yessica's mother is a real-life superhero. As Yessica's primary caretaker, she has been diligent in advocating for her daughter's individualized education, therapies, and care since childhood. High-functioning autism has already primed our superhero for a life of potential struggles and obstacles. Now, new diagnoses of a brain aneurysm and stroke weighed heavy. "I should have brought her in sooner"—a phrase I wish no parent would utter but one I hear all too often. I told her that much like parenting, medicine is an art. Guilt over perceived delays in care bind us to the past, when what we must do is live in the present and move forward. Armed with all the medical knowledge she could soak up, our superhero and her daughter left the hospital. I was certain I would not see them again.

Back at home, I opened Yessica's chart. My first intuition was actually not one of doom. I assumed she was back for a routine angiography, possible re-intervention, and I was looking forward to catching up. I often start my pre-work encounters by reading through my patients' notes, but this time I initially scrolled through her active medication list. My heart sank and I could immediately tell she was critically ill by the new medicines she was on. She went from someone I thought I would never see again to someone I thought may not survive the night. She developed a new aneurysm and bled into her brain. I mentally prepared myself for the worst, to hold her mother's hand and support her through the loss of a child. After getting the full story from my colleague, I started my shift by breaking the news that Yessica would have to undergo an emergent operation to relieve the pressure in her brain. The sounds of her mother wailing and screaming to save her baby still haunt me.

It was touch-and-go, but I spent every waking moment by Yessica's bedside and she survived that night. I was surprised to find out that Yessica's mother remembered me from the prior admission, particularly because it was a short one. I often wonder the impact physicians have on families after they leave the hospital. Did I say the right thing? Did I say enough to convey the important message? Should I have warned her more? Before Yessica's emergent surgery, I told her mother that I was not sure her daughter would be alive by the morning. When I was a trainee, I thought that this kind of honesty was too brutal. But throughout my career, I learned the hard way that anything but this kind of transparency is even more brutal and cruel. I left that morning thinking Yessica's mother now hated me because I was the pessimistic doctor who lied to her and did not have enough faith. I was not looking forward to my next hospital shift.

Over the next several days, I keenly followed Yessica's ICU course from afar. She continued to struggle and was incredibly unstable. My next night shift was finally upon me. I nervously entered the room and saw Yessica's mother fidgeting at the bedside. I spent the next hour talking with her and expressed some optimism that Yessica was still fighting for her life. I jokingly asked if she disliked me for my brutal honesty (I have never asked a parent this, but felt comfortable and connected enough to do so in that moment). Her eyes lit up and she told me, "What? You are my favorite." I was dumbfounded. But with some renewed confidence, my relationship with this superhero mother continued to strengthen over the coming weeks.

Every time she would see me, she would tell the bedside nurse that her favorite doctor was here and we would have a heart to heart. She told me her fears, anxieties, worries, and uncertainties about the future. I listened with an occasional sympathetic shoulder rub. After a while I finally mustered the courage to ask, "Why am I your favorite?" still puzzled by this. She replied, "The first night we got here, I saw in your eyes and heard in your voice that this was the end. But you stayed by my daughter's side the whole time and did not give up. I just trust you." I still did not know what I did to earn so much of her trust; however, I felt even more impassioned to prove to her that I deserved it.

I spent hours a day talking to Yessica's mother and getting to know more of her story. I watched old videos of her spunky daughter, full of life and ambition. Before I examined Yessica, I would always gently caress her arm and tell her everything was going to be okay. One day, her mother finally confided in me that she developed significant post-traumatic stress after losing a close relative. She eventually told me that she was in a situation where the doctors were not upfront about prognosis and wished they were just honest with her. It finally clicked. I have seen doctors so terrified of revealing the truth because of the eventual sobbing, rage, and misguided anger at the clinician. But I have come to realize that this is a natural, reflexive human grief response. Maybe if enough doctors asked parents if they hated them for their honesty, those same terrified doctors would be more inclined to be vulnerable and honest in the future.

As a pediatric intensivist, I meet families and their critically ill children at different points in their life journeys. I see parents of medically complex children and marvel at the intimate knowledge of their child. They become encyclopedias of information, timelines, and nuances. My advice to colleagues is to get to know these parents as individuals beyond their role of caretaker. Be honest with them—they can handle it. Talk to them frequently and get to know their stories. Your actions and words are powerful tools; wield them responsibly. Understand that their journey is a long and complicated one and admissions to the hospital are only a snapshot in time. In fact, this is just the beginning of our superhero mother's long journey. I feel so grateful to be a small part of it because of all the lessons she taught me and the new things I learned about myself. Her daughter will never be the same and she knows it. "I know that this is the new normal. I'm prepared to do whatever it takes. I'm her momma." But, she is more than just a mother. She is a real-life superhero.

Parent Commentary

This doctor's advice to his colleagues as summed up in the last paragraph of his story speaks not only to his colleagues, but also perfectly speaks for the parents of his patients. From a parent's perspective, he nails what we want from our child's doctors: be honest, spend time getting to know us, and understand there is more to our lives than what you see in the hospital. His story shows how communication, honesty, and compassion create trust.

This doctor was surprised that he was this mother's "favorite" because he initially feared that by being honest he would lose her trust. However, I believe there is more than just being honest that creates the trusting relationship with your patient's parent. It is how that honesty is delivered. Honesty can be delivered bluntly, or it can be wrapped in compassion. Yes, the facts regarding our child's condition or prognosis can be brutal; however, when this devastating information is delivered, its impact on the parent can be softened when it is accompanied by compassion and ongoing communication, as this story shares. This doctor showed great compassion in staying by his critically ill patient's side throughout the night—compassion that her mother noticed. He spent time talking with Yessica's mother to get to know her story—not just a few minutes of his time, but hours.

I am not a doctor so I cannot speak to why it would be surprising to a doctor when a parent feels a special connection to them. But what I can say is that we encounter many doctors throughout our child's life, and while they may all be good people and competent clinicians, it is the rare few that we connect with in the way that Yessica's mother connected with this doctor. These connections are invaluable to us as we navigate the challenging (and rewarding) journey of caring for our child. So yes, please be honest, please spend time with us, and get to know our story. These things all create trust and when we trust you, it is almost guaranteed that you will become one of our favorites.

Physician Commentary

Delivering a poor—or "guarded" to put it euphemistically—prognosis (outlook), is one of the most feared moments of the life of a physician who deals with critically ill children. We have developed a vast repertoire of linguistic gymnastics to soften the blow. "Things don't look good." "The outlook is uncertain." And the immortal "I'm very worried." How do we think parents interpret these vagaries? Who are we trying to protect when we couch the truth? I would posit, it is to protect ourselves as much as to protect our patients' parents. Honestly, show me one human being who actually enjoys giving bad news! It is truth and experience—delivered with empathy and compassion—that our parents expect from us.

Having said this, there is very little true science behind developing a prognosis. Every patient is different. The same "injury"—such as a type of brain hemorrhage—in two different patients may portend very different outcomes. In general, the younger the patient, the more "plasticity" or capacity for recovery there may be. Physicians can only provide a reasonable range of expectations, but as was evident from this heartfelt story, there is no substitution for honesty. Honesty can be delivered in many different ways, and when it comes to our most vulnerable children and their families, the only "right" way to deliver honesty is with the utmost of compassion and empathy. There is no cookie cutter approach, and each physician must find their own language. For junior physicians reading this, watch your senior physicians to learn. For experienced physicians, please pass on your wisdom in this realm to your trainees and junior doctors. If medicine is as much art as science, this is where the art really comes in.

Beyond the Numbers

20

There exists a unique feeling of being exposed to direct sunlight after being indoors and awake for over 24 hours. Riding in the back of a car, my colleague and I were on a way to a memorial fundraiser.

Training to become a provider in the Pediatric Intensive Care Unit is both an isolating and a bonding experience. For all those not in this field of medicine, it places the provider on a metaphorical island. It is not a relatable experience, rather one that adds distance to even the deepest rooted of past relationships. For those who share this journey with you, it produces a relationship that cannot be replicated. It was this bond that made my friend get into the car with me and drive over an hour and a half through traffic. The long drive gave us both the ability to reflect on what the loss of this particular patient meant to us.

At the onset of my training, there was such a steep learning curve that patient experiences were often rushed and hurried. Keeping up with admissions as they came, while also progressing patients so they could be transferred out of the unit to maintain bed-space, was an ongoing puzzle that needed solving. As I made my way down the series of rooms, this one room caught my eye. There was a "healthy" looking young man sitting up in bed watching TV. Where cartoons reign supreme, Phil was watching the PGA tour. I took the time to just sit and talk with him. We spoke, not within the confines of the physician-patient relationship, but as golfers. We discussed his interest in sports, TV, movies, and even video games. His parents took me in, not just as a part of his medical team, but as one of his friends. We shared meals together. Phil and his parents were able to shed light into his long-standing battle with cancer. The continuous trips to the hospital for chemotherapy and office visits. Years of infusions, lab draws, and procedures. Yet despite all of his challenges, Phil's uplifting spirit remained unchanged. Even with these recurrent therapies and procedures, he managed to keep his golf swing picture-perfect. There was a magnetism with this family. When I was not working in the ICU, I found myself coming into room six on my spare time to hang out with my buddy. Eventually Phil was discharged from the hospital, the leukemia not cured, but the acute condition resolved.

© Springer Nature Switzerland AG 2021
A. F. Schrooten, B. P. Markovitz, *Shared Struggles*,
https://doi.org/10.1007/978-3-030-68020-6_20

The first year of training passed. I assumed Phil had returned to what was his "normal" life. As I started my time in the ICU again, months down the road I saw Phil's name on my patient list. Even though being in the ICU is never a good place to be, a little part of me was excited to see him and his family. I finished going through my daily numbers and, as I made my way down the hall, I threw on my personal protective equipment and turned into his room. Although it was daytime, the curtains were drawn and there existed a darkness. What I saw was nothing like what my imagination had previously painted.

I saw Phil's mother sitting at his bedside. She feigned a smile, but her face clearly expressed a different story. Eyes so heavy that it seemed like she had just now taken a momentary break from crying. Phil laid motionless in the bed. A BiPAP machine was breathing into his face; he was unable to make any purposeful movements. He just lay there, still. The only noise in the room was that of the BiPAP machine, a whirling of pressurized air going in and out. Internally, I knew that the leukemic cells which were coursing through his veins had finally taken their toll, breaking down the functions of what the healthy cells should be doing. And it showed. If ever an image of hopelessness came to mind, it was that moment in time for me.

Working in critical care medicine, there is an understanding of a patient once you lay eyes on them. There is either an expectation of recovery, having a long-term stay where they are technology reliant or an understanding that they will not be walking out of the hospital. Looking at Phil laying there, it certainly seemed like his would be the latter.

Reflecting back, my colleagues told me the dire circumstances behind Phil's return to the ICU; however, I never truly heard their words. I knew a young man who was strong, driven, motivated, and full of life despite his ongoing disease. In my eyes, all of the warnings of respiratory failure did not apply to him; he could overcome anything. In reality, he was not the same young man. His heart was struggling, albeit beating. His lungs were technically exchanging oxygen and carbon dioxide, but only under the crutch of pressurized air. Motionless. Lifeless.

I spent the next 2 days speaking at length with his family. My attending physician knew the relationship we had and she gave me the autonomy to have the difficult discussions. Phil's condition truly had worsened. He wound up on a ventilator with no hope for alternative chemotherapy agents. Every organ in his body was deteriorating and I had to sit across from his family and describe to them the hopelessness of the situation. This family who took me in as their own and provided me with meals when I did not have the opportunity to feed myself amidst the work. I was the one who had to tell them that the treatment had reached a point of futility. Sitting across from this defeated family and expressing these points, I felt like I was extinguishing any last hope they had for the recovery of their son. As they wept, I joined alongside. I knew my buddy was not meant for this world. He was removed from life support surrounded by his mother, father, and brother. The family left the hospital after saying goodbye. I knew that somewhere in the universe they continued to exist, but in a world that they probably no longer understood.

As I approached my third and final year of my ICU training, I was surprised to see an email about a memorial golf tournament in Phil's honor. Although the date of the tournament meant that I would need to stay awake after already being awake for 30 hours, it would not be a deterrent. All these memories ran through my sleepless mind on the drive. I had no idea what emotions would run through me when I saw Phil's family. Would they be upset that I was as direct as I was with them during our final conversations? Would I bring the emotions of Phil's loss rushing back? Was this really a good idea for me to show my face? A nervous energy took over me as we approached the clubhouse.

As I was writing my name down at the registration table, I heard a familiar voice and turned around. She was smiling and crying simultaneously. Phil's mother called over her family and introduced them to me. They all knew of me and hugged me as if I was a member of the family. When I finally had the chance to speak to Phil's mother and father, they looked back on their time in the hospital and especially the ICU. For all the anguish and suffering they had to endure, there also existed brief moments of reprieve when we all just hung out together. For them, I was not the bearer of bad news, but rather the trusted friend who wanted the best for their son.

I sit at my computer, 4 years later, looking back at the memories from this encounter. It hurt. A lot. I carry the pain of Phil's passing to this date. It enlightened me to just what this field does to us. We are put in charge of the worst part of a person's life. In this time, we must establish trust between each other. This trust can easily be a one-way street where the credentials behind the name of a physician can just be taken as the guiding force for patient management. This was one of my first instances where a personal connection with a patient was made. In Phil, I saw a younger version of myself and it produced a friendship.

Where I thought that I could partition the work of a physician and a friend, it turns out that these two can work hand in hand. It should not be a forced relationship, however, when that connection feels natural it should be cultivated. This field cannot just be about blood pressures, heart rates, and oxygen saturations. There exists a human nature to patient connection beyond the numbers that should also be fostered. Within this realm, the potential for pain exists, but so too does the potential to learn about the human who is being supported by the machine.

Parent Commentary

As a parent who has formed friendships with my son's doctors, it is heartwarming to read this story from a young doctor. I could not agree more that it is okay to be both a doctor and friend with your patient (or your patient's parent) when the connection feels natural. As with any relationship, moving from a doctor-patient relationship to a doctor-patient-friend relationship is not without emotional risks. This doctor wept with his patient's family; he carried a heavier burden when he had to tell them there were no more treatment options for their son. He did not have to put himself in a situation that would cause him to so personally and deeply feel the grief his patient's family was going through. Understandably, most doctors do not. Perhaps he did not know that his natural connection with his patient and resulting friendship would come at a greater emotional cost than if he had kept the relationship with his patient strictly formal. However, he does not regret his decision, he honors it. And going forward with the lessons he learned from this experience, his patients and their parents are all the more fortunate to come under his compassionate care.

This doctor was worried about the reaction he would receive from Phil's parents when they saw him years after their son's death. He need not have been. The fear that your presence or words might stir up the painful emotions surrounding our child's death is unnecessary. We never forget the pain, however, with time, the pain softens and we remember with gratitude the people who were present with us during the most difficult time in our lives. We want to be reminded that our child is remembered by their doctor. We want to be reminded that you were there, that you cared, and that you grieved with us. The honesty and compassion shown by our child's doctor will always soften the pain of the circumstances that brought us all together in the first place. The greater the connection we feel with our child's doctor, the greater the trust—a trust we cherish and carry with us long after the doctor-patient relationship has ended.

Physician Commentary

This story strikes deeply to critical care physicians, or it should. For reasons beyond our reckoning, we form bonds, far beyond the venerated physician-patient (or physician-family) "therapeutic relationship" with some patients and families. Physicians must earn the trust of their patients and families; it is not a given. There are many avenues to establish this bond, but they all come down to empathy.

Sadly, in our usual world in the ICU of fast-paced critical decisions and invasive interventions, physicians rarely have the time to bond to patients and families as this physician was able to achieve. In this case, a love of sports (golf in particular) enabled this connection. It sounds like the physician, patient, and family truly came to know one another as just people, with hopes, dreams, interests, and likes. These connections are truly special, to be cherished, as was evidently clear in how this physician writes in this story. Even if we do not go outside the typical "medical" relationship with our patients, we can and should view each child, each family, as unique, with their own values and goals. Physicians should afford, within the limits possible, patients and families the widest latitude in decision-making at critical moments in the course of their disease.

At the same time, critical care physicians have to maintain a balance of empathy and self-protection. This is not easy to say. If physicians were as deeply impacted by the passing of every one of our patients as this one was, it would be hard to stay on course. In pediatric critical care, we are fortunate, compared to our colleagues caring for adults, that only 3-5% of our patients die. But in the course of a career, that can represent dozens, or hundreds of deaths. Each death should weigh heavily upon us, but if it weighs too heavily, our ability to care for the 95% of patients that survive, and to shepherd those destined to die to a dignified end, can be compromised. For critical care physicians, finding this balance of connection, empathy, and resilience to care for the next child, is a hallmark of our professional lives.

Shared Experience

21

As I watched a tear crawl down Lisa's cheek, I saw fear. Her beautiful 1-month-old son, Michael, had started seizing uncontrollably the night before and was admitted to the Pediatric Intensive Care Unit (PICU). Just before I walked into Michael's room the next morning, he had finally stopped seizing. However, this reprieve in her son's seizures did not relieve the fear that consumed Lisa's every move. I could sense her fear of the unknown, fear of the known, fear of disappointment, fear of ignorance, fear of knowledge, fear of being alone, fear of the people around her, fear of speaking up, and fear of remaining silent.

My fellow told me that Lisa was upset and angry about her interactions with the hospital and health care team. After Michael's first seizure several weeks ago, he was sent home from the hospital with a monitor to alert Lisa if he stopped breathing in his sleep from a seizure. Beyond that, Lisa was given little information on how to take care of her son. She was also told that the first available appointment with a neurologist was 3 months away.

As Lisa reached over to adjust Michael's soft blanket, I wondered how much of myself I should share in my efforts to help her face these fears that now surfaced as, arguably, justifiable anger. Michael had only been home and seizure-free for a few weeks when Lisa saw the familiar stare in his eyes, followed by a dance of body twitches. She called the neurologist as she had been instructed. When an hour passed without a call back, Lisa dialed 9-1-1 and Michael was transported to the hospital. The emergency department physician attempted to contact Michael's neurologist, only to get the on-duty physician, who, having never met Michael, gave the standard management advice. After the medications took effect and the seizures stopped, Lisa and Michael found themselves back in the now familiar PICU.

I wondered how much of the PICU was reminiscent of home's dark places—the lack of sleep, lack of confidence in Michael's care plan, and lack of certainty about what comes next. By now she had trained her body to react to each beep of the monitors. After all, it was this response to Michael's home monitor that would ensure her readiness should an emergent need arise. Like home, where false alarms leave Lisa in a constant hyperaware and anxious state, the seemingly continuous beeping of monitors in the PICU only served to maintain her sleep-deprived state and remind her of the constant, uncontrolled peril swirling around her son and his future.

I had not met Lisa before this PICU admission, but I had seen those expressions of fear, anger, and lack of control on the faces of many parents in the PICU. However, as I examined Michael and discussed my thoughts about the care plan for the day, it was my brother's face that came to mind. I saw in my mind's eye my brother's face as he watched his 6-year-old son, who also suffers with seizures, struggle to tie his shoes, a task which he had once mastered. I saw my brother's face as he recounted the neurologist's plan to remix the concoction of prescribed poisons—what we call medicine—with seemingly little logic and only limited consideration of his son's unique situation. I saw my brother's face as he wrapped his young son's head with a homemade monitor developed to alarm if he seized during the night. I saw my brother's face of today, as his son moves into adolescence. Although his son has managed to relearn to tie his shoes and the homemade monitor rarely alarms, my brother's face still reflects fear of an uncertain future and questions about how life as an adult will unfold for his son.

As I looked at Lisa and saw my brother, I wrestled to choose my words. Ironic, since I am a teacher of words. In my work and my teaching, I preach the importance of talking to parents of seriously ill children with empathy when giving bad news and trying to provide support. Yet, as I looked at Lisa's face, I wondered what that meant for me in this particular situation.

Author Brené Brown eloquently describes the keys to responding empathetically: (1) taking the perspective of another person; (2) not judging; (3) recognizing emotion; and (4) communicating what you observe. She talks of "feeling with people" and connecting with something inside yourself that knows the feelings or experiences of others. So I found myself struggling with how much of myself, my family, and what I have seen to reveal as I try to connect with Lisa.

Frankly, my personal and professional life have become so strangely and inexorably connected that sometimes I wonder where one stops and the other begins. For 9 months, I walked across the bridge connecting the Children's Hospital to the adult hospital multiple times a week, sometimes daily, for my own cancer treatment. I would leave work for chemotherapy, radiation, physical therapy, or whatever the appointment of the day was. After my appointment, I would cross back over the bridge and get back to work. Although the most intense parts of my treatment are done, appointments remain regular and frequent. As new challenges emerge, I still make that now familiar walk which blends my work life with my personal challenges.

I know I am not the only doctor whose perspective changes after a significant life event. I often hear colleagues talk about how they see their pediatric patients in a new light after having kids of their own. Still, when I find myself in front of parents like Lisa, I wonder if, in my effort to connect and feel what Lisa feels, in my efforts to be empathetic, I should expose my own wave of emotions. I wonder if sharing personal information helps or selfishly detracts. After all, it is not about me. I would certainly not want anyone to interpret my sharing personal information as a surrogate for claiming to know how they feel. I rarely share anything about what I or my brother have gone through with the parents of the children I care for. With Lisa, I could not resist.

When I mentioned that I have a nephew with an unexplained seizure disorder, I could see Lisa's entire body soften just a bit. As I shared how my brother struggles with fears about what might happen to his son during the night, I could sense her tense muscles relaxing. When I mentioned that I too found it complicated and exhausting to find a doctor who I trusted, Lisa actually felt comfortable enough to step away from Michael's crib and sit down with me. When I shared that I worry daily about the future for my nephew and myself, I could feel in myself a sense of community with Lisa. I think she felt it also.

I know that I do not have to experience everything my patients and families go through to have empathy. I also know I did not take away all of Lisa's fears in those moments. Maybe I did not even take away any of her fears. However, I think by sharing a bit of myself, Lisa knew that I had heard her and that on some level I was trying to feel a bit of what she was feeling. I hope that for at least a few moments Lisa realized that she was not alone.

Parent Commentary

Being in the hospital with your sick child is a very lonely experience, especially in the intensive care unit where you are isolated behind closed glass doors. We see the doctors, nurses, and other staff members coming and going as we look through the glass barrier that separates "us" from "them." Sometimes we cannot help but feel envious and angry that they get to go home at the end of their shift, leaving their work and the struggles of their patients behind. We tell ourselves that they do not understand. We assume they go home to their healthy kids and the life we wish we were living.

By sharing her own story, this doctor reminds us that sick children and hardships do not discriminate. Empathy is the ability to understand and share the feelings of others. This doctor had some understanding of what Michael's mother was going through because of her brother and nephew. She acknowledged that she rarely shares personal information with parents, but in this case, she sensed that sharing her experience would be helpful for Michael's mother. She was right.

Doctors are humans just like the rest of us. However, whether it is because of what they are taught in medical school and training or what they personally believe is right, doctors seem to be reluctant to reveal the human side of themselves. They often keep their encounter with parents at arm's length and limited to an exchange of information. Certainly, there are professional boundaries that doctors have to respect, but doctors are not blank slates. Like the rest of us, they all have personal experiences that make up who they are. Through sharing information about themselves that is appropriate for the patient and parent in front of them, they reveal themselves as human beings, not merely conveyors of information.

In those rare cases when our child's doctor has a personal understanding of what we are going through, by sharing their own experiences it helps mitigate the "us" versus "them" feeling and, as Michael's mother illustrated, this human connection can lift the tremendous weight that comes from feeling alone and not understood. Parents want to see and know the human side of doctors. This connection creates a space for trust and communication, which is especially important in the long-term relationships we have with many of our child's doctors.

Physician Commentary

This is a delicate balance that many physicians face: how much, if anything, to reveal of their own lives in an effort to establish a bond with families. Physicians should never, ever state the equivalent of: "I know what you are going through." But revealing a small part of ourselves or our own struggles, at the right moment, with the right family, can indeed be powerful. I wish I had a formula to propose for when this is, or is not appropriate. I do not.

Empathy, however, is a universal connection mechanism that can create a bond, even without a shared experience. The opposite of empathy is shame, as the author appropriately cites Brené Brown. Empathy smothers shame. Unstated in many of these stories is shame. Parents wonder what they did wrong to bring this "sentence" upon their child and themselves. It is not logical, but it is human to think this way. Physicians, by creating an empathic connection with their patients and families, can help wash away this feeling. This physician recognized, intuitively, the need to make this connection. However, it does not always take having a similar medical situation in one's family to make this connection.

Tying the Thread into a Bond

22

My mother was a pediatrician—an old-fashioned, old-school, solo practitioner who practiced for over 40 years on the Southside of Chicago. She cared for multigenerational families, intimately delivering care that fostered genuine, life-long relationships. Her career ran so deep she spent her final years treating the grandchildren of patients she looked after as infants.

Going into critical care pediatrics, I recognized I would not have the same longitudinal relationships with my patients. But my mother's story gave me the necessary insight to compress that impact of care into some of the most poignant and meaningful days any family could experience. What I gave up in length, I gained in depth. That type of interaction works perfectly with my personality, capitalizing on the rapid-fire, sometimes passing, often necessarily "short attention span" ICU environment. Sharing the intensity and depth of a moment with families in my care defined every memorable relationship throughout my career. However, some patients manage to transcend those isolated impactful moments, leading to lasting relationships that constantly remind me of my purpose as a pediatrician, caregiver, and father.

One such relationship started while working with the family of an infant, Anna, with a critical heart defect, an anomalous origin of the left coronary artery. While life-threatening, the defect has a straightforward surgical correction and a historically good outcome, usually leading to a long and healthy life. Of course, we all know historical outcomes cannot always predict the future. Unfortunately for her case, heart damage prior to surgery left Anna with such poor function that a transplant was necessary.

The days between the diagnosis, surgery, and unfavorable fallout quickly swelled to desperation after numerous complications—from cardiac arrests, to sudden deteriorations, even to multi-organ injury. During our shared ride on this chaotic emotional rollercoaster, I joined a family in their most vulnerable moments. Facing those moments with confidence, kindness, and care ultimately define careers like my own; I understand that this is my true calling. While the complications brought constant intensity, nothing compared to the decision to move forward with transplantation. Her family understood that though cardiac transplantation is lifesaving,

© Springer Nature Switzerland AG 2021
A. F. Schrooten, B. P. Markovitz, *Shared Struggles*,
https://doi.org/10.1007/978-3-030-68020-6_22

it effectively trades one disease for another—an acute threat for a chronic concern. Transplantation requires management, respect, and monitoring. During the listing process, Anna's parents clearly struggled with the decision to set their baby daughter on the best path. Should they commit to a lifetime of struggle with an uncertain outcome, or should they hang on to a slight chance of medically managed heart failure? Ultimately, they chose to list for transplantation.

As fate would have it, just several hours later an organ became available, and the donor was local. The original recipient had to emergently refuse the organ while the team was already performing the donor operation. This situation allowed for the right of first refusal for the local hospital, putting Anna one on the list. But that meant her parents had to make a decision fast or the organ would go to the next patient.

Time became compressed.

I was not even on clinical service that day. I just happened to be in the CICU the hour these events transpired. I found Anna's mother alone, her husband home caring for their other children across the state. During that time, the entire care team rallied around her for support, but they still could not make a decision for her. So, as she heavily debated the future of her infant daughter, she turned to me for guidance.

Her struggle unfolded in front of me. The struggle with a decision that impacted the life of her child, her family, and herself. There really was no going back once the decision was made; and she fully understood that fact. Our conversation initially revolved around statistics, outcomes, and data. This is a conversation I felt comfortable with because it was based in the science of medicine. However, it inevitably took a much more personal tone as data gave way to emotion. Finally, she asked me to tell her what I would do in this situation. Ultimately, she asked me to tell her what to do.

As a pediatrician, we are often faced with the question, "What would you do if this was your child?" I have to admit, I hate it. Throughout my career, I hid behind a façade of detachment: it is not my child and I should separate myself to give genuinely objective advice. I also never wanted to actually think about a reality where my own son was in such a painful situation. So, in that moment with that confused, desperate mother, I learned that the "distance" I used as protection had to be removed. I needed to think clearly and empathetically for someone who simply could not under the mounting pressure. As I told her to take the heart, I learned the most important lesson of my career: allow yourself to be vulnerable. Bridge the distance between patient and provider. Allow yourself to cross the imaginary line of somehow exerting undue influence. I have heard that approach referred to as the ideal of "detached concern." Many of us have been taught that emotions can interfere with making objective diagnoses and remaining scientific. We were told that we must serve as an impartial moral agent who is able to care for all types of patients. That has changed for me.

I have spent the rest of my career explaining to trainees that anyone can turn the right knobs on a ventilator or change delivery rates of inotropes, but a doctor's true colors show in moments spent guiding a family through the most difficult situations in their lives. In moments like these, the job becomes more than a profession or even a calling; it becomes a sacred covenant—a pledge to share in the care of another individual.

Anna was successfully transplanted that day. After recovery, she was discharged and did very well for years. Life went on. Soon, I left my position at that institution, and my family and I moved to a new city. Yet despite the distance, I stayed in contact with Anna's family, swapping letters and the occasional social media post. One year, the family shared a special ornament with me, forever making Christmas a special time of remembrance. Hanging that ornament as the last decoration on the tree every year, now a tradition in my household, constantly reminded me of a meaningful, life-long relationship, one that deeply impacted me despite the supposed impersonal dealings of an ICU.

The overwhelming majority of patients who experience an ICU leave our world as quickly and permanently as they came in. This is really what a physician like me is supposed to do. However, in the world of modern medicine, and especially in my subspecialty of cardiac critical care, ICUs often readmit previous patients, as they return for more surgeries or interventions. They require repeat care for infectious complications or even trauma. However, regardless of the cause, patient and physician paths cross more frequently than ever. Even through the uncertain call and service schedules, the ships passing in the night occasionally find one another and embrace like old friends.

From this relationship and the countless repeat interactions with families, I grew to appreciate the unique dynamics of ICU relationships. Every moment with a family—from the briefest encounters, to the most impactful memories—serves a deep role in the lives of everyone involved. Each of these interactions ties a life-long thread between the physician and the patient and their family. While an ICU career may often cut those threads short or pull them out seemingly at random, it still creates deeply personal, unbreakable bonds. Those bonds can take many forms and many durations, but they remain the core foundation to the essence of being a physician.

Parent Commentary

We have all had to make decisions in our life where the outcome could not be guaranteed. However, few of us (fortunately) have been asked to make decisions where the consequences determine whether our child lives or dies. I have not personally been in a situation where I have asked a doctor "what would you do?" when I had to a make a medical decision for my son. However, I have certainly asked the doctors I trust for their opinions. We all want reassurance from the doctors who have the experience and expertise we do not have.

In general, doctors make decisions based on their education and experience and parents make decisions based on their "gut." (Not to suggest that parents do not incorporate their knowledge of their child's condition and treatment options or that doctors do not incorporate their intuition.) Parents acquire their "gut" or parental intuition over time and with experience. When I was first thrust into the world of medical complexity, rare diseases, and medical technology, I was completely lost and uncertain. My child was a newborn; I had no experience with him, his medical condition, medical technology, or the plethora of medical subspecialties we encountered. I had no gut feelings when it came to making decisions for my son, except that I wanted him to live. With time and experience, my parental intuition developed and became something I could trust. Experienced parents who are often faced with difficult decisions regarding their medically complex child place a lot of weight on what "feels" right to them.

In this story, you have a parent who had to make a life or death decision for her infant daughter, and the decision had to be made quickly and without her husband's presence. Her child had a complicated heart condition that did not follow the "rules." She did not yet have years of experience as the parent of a child with a complex heart disease and no roadmap to follow. I can understand this parent being in a place where she wanted someone to tell her what to do. I imagine she wanted someone to help carry the burden of the decision with her. I can also understand why a doctor does not like being placed in that position. It is a heavy burden to carry. I think it was courageous for this doctor to go against his preference to steer clear of answering that question. He saw a mother who desperately wanted help and he honored her feelings over his own. In this case, the decision chosen was the right one because it had a successful outcome. But what if it had not? That is the risk. I am certain those parents who ask the question, "what would you do?" are forever grateful for those doctors who take the risk and answer it.

Physician Commentary

"What would you do doctor if this was your child?" These are the ten most feared words in Pediatrics in general, and in pediatric complex or intensive care patients in particular. The truthful answer should be: "I have no idea." Because we do not. (Of course, there is always the incredibly rare chance a pediatrician actually did have to make such a decision about their own child with the same condition at the same time, but this is extraordinarily rare.) As much as we talk—even in this book—about empathizing with parents, putting yourselves in their shoes, understand their values—this is simply not a fair question. I may have a glimpse of what the parent in front of me is going through with their child, but to make it my child creates two problems.

First, we truly have no way to predict how we would behave in the exact situation the parent in front of us is facing were the child really our own. Do you know exactly how you would behave in an earthquake? If you saw a horrible tragedy play itself out in front of you? We simply cannot predict a hypothetical future, especially when being asked about our own children. The second problematic issue with this question is raised elsewhere in this book: if I even could answer this question, I would be—by definition—applying my own values, heritage, and beliefs to bear. The last thing a physician should do is impose their own value systems on their patients' families. This is a core moral principle for physicians to uphold.

What this question does, in my opinion, is to allow physicians to tell the parents what they think the right thing to do is for the child in front of them. But it is somewhat disingenuous to offer your professional opinion (which is not only acceptable to do but is morally incumbent for a physician to do) in the guise of pretending to know what you would do if this were your own child. This question can and should be answered, something like this:

"I can't begin to imagine how I would behave in this situation. I just don't know. But what I can tell you, based on our discussions of your hopes and values for your child, and my medical knowledge and experience, I recommend we embark on treatment plan B…" Of course this answer presupposes the physician has, indeed, discussed the family's hopes, values, and goals, which absolutely must be done before answering such value-laden questions.

Part III

Communication

The single biggest problem in communication is the illusion that it has taken place. –George Bernard Shaw

A Voice That Doesn't Use Words

23

"There is a voice that doesn't use words. Listen." —Rumi.

"Frequent flyer," the Pediatric Intensive Care (PICU) Fellow said with a sigh, giving me a heads-up on the patient who would soon be arriving from the Emergency Department (ED). "Usual drill. Might as well get a head start and call the usual list of consults—cardiology, neurology, pulmonology, endocrinology. It's always the same thing—at least once a month she's admitted all out of whack, we straighten her out and tidy things up, send her home. Until the next time."

I was moonlighting weekends in the PICU for some extra cash, having just started my pediatric palliative care fellowship. I was still getting used to the institution, its workflow and culture, though in most ways it was pretty similar to all the other places I had trained and worked as a physician. And I was already familiar with the concept of the "frequent flyer"; enough so that even without knowing this patient's actual diagnosis or specific reason for admission, I was pretty sure I could conjure up a solid mental image of the admission I was about to do. I had admitted dozens, if not hundreds, of so-called frequent flyers in my training and early career, and felt like I had the routine down. These kids typically had some variety of complex chronic illness, an umbrella term for conditions that often involved multiple organ systems, long lists of medications, and often some form of technology dependence (e.g., feeding tubes, tracheostomies, BiPAP).

This particular young woman was no exception. Maybe early teens (though hard to tell just by appearance), with a rare metabolic syndrome that I thought I remembered reading about once but really knew nothing about. She arrived in the PICU on the transport bed curled up on her side, blanket tangled around her feet. Her arms and legs seemed to be tightly contracted at every joint possible (twisted like a human pretzel, I thought to myself, though I now recall that with shame). Her bulging eyes locked intensely on something off to the side, though it was not at all clear that she was looking at anything specific; she did not appear to be responding to, or even aware of, her surroundings.

© Springer Nature Switzerland AG 2021
A. F. Schrooten, B. P. Markovitz, *Shared Struggles*,
https://doi.org/10.1007/978-3-030-68020-6_23

She was accompanied by her mother, a harried-looking woman, maybe in her 40's but with a deeply lined face and graying hair up in a messy bun. As they rolled into the PICU the mother kept pace at the side of the bed, halfway bent over the rail, speaking quietly with her daughter, and massaging one contorted shoulder.

The admission process itself went more or less as expected: the patient (who I learned from a glance at the ED papers was named Cassie[1]) was transferred to a PICU bed and the nurse busily went about arranging the various bedding, tubes, and wires she would need to monitor and maintain comfort. While this was going on, I quickly perused the electronic record (dozens of seemingly identical admissions that, if it were not for slightly different lab values I would have said were cut and pasted by past clinicians). Once Cassie was more or less settled in bed (still contracted at all joints and lying on her side, but now under a tidy white sheet), I took a brief history from her mom, having already more or less decided on the best path forward. As she described the past several days of low fevers and increased seizure activity, I was already mentally composing orders and lists of necessary consult services.

Having moved on to a cursory physical exam, I was just finishing up auscultating the awkward contours of her back when her mom, now facing both me and Cassie on the opposite side of the bed, looked at me and said, "Cassie's actually a bit hungry now."

What? I asked, pulling the stethoscope from my ears.

"She's hungry. Her feeds were held down in the ED, which she didn't really care about down there, but now she wants them."

I stood, looping the stethoscope over my neck like a prizefighter's belt. Well, I explained, I would like to continue holding off on feeds for now, at least until we have a better idea of what is going on. It would be safer to just stick with IV fluids for at least the next few hours.

"Not a good idea," she said, shaking her head. "I don't know if it's the antibiotics, or the fever is down, or if it's the fluids she got downstairs, but she's feeling better. She just told me she's hungry, which she never does unless she's feeling okay."

Over mom's shoulder I caught a glimpse of the bedside nurse's face. She rolled her eyes and winked at me.

Sorry, I said, I must not have heard her. I moved around to the foot of the bed to get a better look at Cassie, but as far as I could see her face was frozen in the same inscrutable rictus as when she had arrived.

"Well, she didn't say it out loud," she explained, sounding a bit annoyed. "She rarely actually says any words. But she communicates with me mostly through her face and eyes. And she just gave me the sort of lip and tongue movement plus blinking that she uses to tell me she's hungry."

Got it, I thought. I could not decide which was less likely, that Cassie actually *ever* vocalized any words or that she had actually just blinked, let alone had done so in a meaningful way to signal hunger. Well, I said, playing for time, let me go run

---

[1] Identifying details have been changed.

things by the fellow and attending, both of whom may be more familiar than I am with Cassie, and I will circle back with a plan.

She looked unhappy, though whether it was worry about her daughter, unhappiness with me, or just her baseline weariness I could not tell. Not caring to find out which, I hurried off to find my colleagues.

The day finished uneventfully, both for me and for Cassie. Cassie indeed got her feeds (after some pushing on her mom's part), and settled in to her "routine" admission. I headed off at the end of my shift, and by the time I returned for another moonlighting shift later that month, Cassie had been discharged home.

Over the next few months, I saw her again a few times during subsequent admissions that happened to overlap with my moonlighting shifts. Each time it seemed like more or less the same thing: a few days of antibiotics, adjustment of antiepileptics and correction of electrolytes, maybe some slight worsening of "baseline" respiratory status, and then discharged back to home. Cassie's mom was, to her credit, clearly devoted to her care. Always at the bedside, always attentive to her needs. But I also learned that she was viewed by the staff as a bit of a kook, albeit a sad and sympathetic kook, always reporting that "Cassie wants this" or "Cassie says that," whereas nobody ever saw Cassie so much as bat an eye.

Months passed, and as I progressed through my palliative care fellowship, I learned a great deal about communication, about listening, about paying attention to parents and children, and keeping their values at the center of the story. But I do not think I ever really connected those lessons with my experience caring for Cassie. That was, until I was told that I would be joining two other palliative care providers for a home visit to see Cassie and her mom.

Home visits were very much not a part of why I went into medicine. My focus had always been much more on the care of children with serious illness in the hospital and clinic settings. As far as I was concerned, home care was this vague entity, composed of services like nursing and hospice care, neither of which I fully understood. And, knowing what I did about Cassie's barely responsive state and her (to me) offbeat mom, it was with some reluctance that I joined my palliative care colleagues for the visit. I grudgingly headed out one cold morning for the hour-long drive to her home, mostly expecting just a wasted morning.

Their modest home, tucked away in a rural wooded area down a dirt road, was a revelation. When we pulled into the driveway and got out of the car, I took my time, hanging back a bit, I suppose hoping to delay even for a few moments my entry into what I assumed would be an awkward visit. But as the front door opened up ahead of me, we were welcomed warmly by Cassie's mom, who radiated energy in a way that I had never seen in the hospital. She brightly offered me tea and gave me a tour of the home, sharing how nice it was to see me outside the hospital after so many PICU visits. Had it really been that many visits, I wondered? Or did she and I just experience time in the PICU differently?

And the home: where I had expected dark, poorly ventilated rooms with shades drawn, instead I found a warm, clean house, brightly lit, with sunlight coming through the many windows, and decorated with a colorful mid-century vibe. Just the sort of place I could have imagined myself living someday! Instead of feeling somber, the place felt alive.

Cassie's homecare nurse, one of two who switched off shifts during the week, seemed delighted to meet me. I had heard her name of course during discussions leading up to past hospital discharges, but she had always been this nebulous figure, part of Cassie's "other," almost imaginary, life. And I suppose that may have been who I was to her as well. But now here she was, in the flesh, eager to show me to Cassie's room. It was on the ground floor and at first glance just felt like a regular, albeit somewhat crowded, child's bedroom. The walls were papered with a light floral pattern, the floor covered with an immaculately vacuumed periwinkle rug, and here too light streamed in through a large window looking out on the woods behind the house. The center of the room was occupied by a large hospital bed, the head surrounded by various medical devices and pumps. The dresser at the side of the room had a few dolls and childish knick-knacks on top, but a couple of drawers left ajar revealed that it had been repurposed to hold equipment: suction, oxygen, extra tubing, syringes, and nasogastric tubes.

At the center of it all, lying in bed under neat floral sheets, was Cassie herself. Much as in the hospital, she appeared to be lying curled up on one side, her gaze fixed out the window. I moved around to where I could see her face, and was struck at once by how peaceful she looked, not at all like she usually did during hospital admissions. I gave her a cheery "hello!", of course feeling that it was more for the benefit of her mom and her nurse than out of any expectation that she would register my presence (let alone know who I was). Then, in a moment that seemed almost staged, she shifted her eyes, looked right at me, and smiled.

I do not want to overstate this. She did not sit up, did not start chatting with me, did not reach for my hand. But for all the times I had seen Cassie in the hospital, this was the first time I had seen a flicker of the person that her mother saw. For the first time it dawned on me (again, with some shame in retrospect at admitting this), that Cassie really did communicate with her mother, and that although she may not have communicated in a way that the rest of the medical team would normally be alert to, it was nonetheless real and purposeful. Sadly, I realized, because I had not been open to the possibility, had not been attuned to the fact that Cassie might have indeed been telling her mom things like "I'm hungry," I had made assumptions about both Cassie and her mom. I do not believe that I had ever treated her as less than a person, but I do believe that I had not left space for her voice, regardless of what "voice" actually meant.

That moment of contact, of connection and real communication with this *person*, remains a pivotal moment in my career. My career is still focused on the care of seriously ill children, many of whom have complex chronic illness. Many of them are neurologically impaired, to the extent that they cannot verbalize language, write, or even signal in a way that a stranger would identify as having meaning. And some of them may very well not have an ability to communicate in any way, or even an awareness of my presence. But many of them do. I always take care now to allow for space for children to express their voice, in whatever form that might take. To not expect that communication occur on my terms, but rather to be open to whatever terms and means of communication, no matter how subtle, a child might choose.

Parent Commentary

This story is one that every parent of a severely disabled, nonverbal child wishes every doctor who cared for their child could read and learn from. I have great respect for this physician's honesty and humility. His initial feelings regarding Cassie's ability to communicate and her mother's ability to interpret what she was communicating are reactions that parents of nonverbal children experience time and time again. We recognize that we are sometimes viewed as delusional or in denial. The fact is, not only can we sense what our nonverbal child is communicating, we can also sense what medical professionals feel about us and our child. If we learn anything from our nonverbal child, it is a keen sense of awareness of nonverbal cues, regardless of who they are coming from.

A parent's first experience learning to communicate with their child is when they bring their newborn baby home from the hospital. All newborn babies—healthy or otherwise communicate without words. As a parent bonds with their baby, we instinctively know what our baby's cry is communicating. We learn to distinguish between a hunger cry, a tired cry, and a not feeling well cry. This parental instinct that allows us to understand our newborn baby only deepens and becomes more highly attuned over the years as we intimately care for our disabled child in every aspect of their lives. No one questions that a baby can communicate through their cries, smiles, and big bright eyes. The same holds true for our disabled child. We have learned to interpret our nonverbal child's gaze, smile, gestures, and nuances. Trust that we know our child and listen to us—we are their voice.

Our child's brain scan, disease, and disability are not determinative of their ability to communicate. If every physician would take the time to pause, look, and read the face and eyes of a nonverbal child, I am almost certain that they will have a moment of connection just as the physician in this story did. My son had a t-shirt with these words printed on it that sum up the important take-away from this story: "Just because I can't talk doesn't mean I have nothing to say."

Physician Commentary

Every physician who cares for children with severe conditions that impair their ability to communicate should not just read this story, they should memorize it. As physicians have learned to recite the muscles in the arm or the chambers in the heart, they should be able to tell this story over and over again.

Although I have not been afforded the opportunity (would I have taken the chance if it was offered?) to visit a patient's home as in this story, I have learned over the years that parents can "read" their nonverbal children with a skill set no physician possesses. I try to imagine that it is simply a different language that is being spoken between child and parent, one that I never learned and never will. Just as we learn to trust our hospital's interpreters to communicate with families who do not speak English, we must treat the parents as interpreters for these children. But these "interpreters" did not take a course to learn the language, they have lived it and learned it over time, often over years. Just as I would never second guess where a cardiac surgeon decides where to cut or how to stitch, who am I to question the person with the most expertise in the world at communication with a nonverbal child?

There is another aspect of this story that merits commentary. This physician describes what could be interpreted as an apparently cold and heartless attitude toward children who are hospitalized frequently: the "frequent flyers." There is truth to this terminology but allow me to suggest that these comments do not necessarily somehow dehumanize these patients or their parents. Physicians are people too, who can be moved by sadness and may build up walls or defenses for emotional protection. We can experience extreme pain to see a child return again and again to the hospital, and project our values and emotions; how terrible this child's life must be to be hospitalized so frequently. Although we may use such terms as jargon and shorthand, it does not mean we necessarily treat these children or their parents with less respect or compassion. Cassie's story also teaches up that these children can and do have meaningful lives outside the hospital, bringing joy to themselves and their families. Perhaps physicians should indeed make house calls once again. With the explosion of the use (finally!) of telemedicine, this is a very realistic and hopeful opportunity.

Brave the Difficult Conversation

24

Keyan spent more days in the hospital than at home during the first 6 years of her life. She is one of quadruplet girls, born at 27 weeks into my pregnancy. During an ultrasound at 25 weeks it was discovered that the blood flow to Keyan's umbilical cord was compromised. We had to make a decision: either let her die in utero or deliver all four babies to save her.

After much thought, prayer, and with hope, we decided to take a risk on all four babies to save Keyan. All four girls spent time in the Neonatal ICU, but Keyan is the only one with chronic health issues. No one really knows if Keyan's health is complicated due to prematurity, if she was compromised in utero, or if her complications are from a brain bleed in the first weeks of her life. It is likely a combination of all three. Keyan lives with cerebral palsy, chronic lung disease, seizures, dysmobility of her gastrointestinal (GI) system, severe visual impairment, and many other conditions that affect her day-to-day living.

Keyan gets all her nutrition from IV nutrition (TPN) administered through a broviac central line placed in her chest. For years, she was in a cycle of septic infection after septic infection with various other infections scattered in between. Her gut leaked bacteria and fungus into her blood stream and the central line aided in the spread of the infected blood. Her GI system deteriorated enough that it complicated her body function well beyond what we ever thought possible. Things were not moving in a good direction. I could feel it in my heart, yet no one on Keyan's care team wanted to talk about it. The focus was always on resolving the immediate problem at hand.

It was in this cycle of infections when Keyan started seeing a pediatric physiatrist from the rehabilitation hospital down the road from our Children's Hospital. Keyan was receiving intensive inpatient therapy at the rehab hospital to regain her strength and endurance after suffering a series of major seizures that left her unable to hold her head up or sit on her own. While at the rehab hospital, Keyan was transferred to Children's Hospital because of another septic central line infection.

© Springer Nature Switzerland AG 2021
A. F. Schrooten, B. P. Markovitz, *Shared Struggles*,
https://doi.org/10.1007/978-3-030-68020-6_24

Early one morning, the physiatrist knocked on the door of Keyan's hospital room. I was surprised to see him, not expecting he would follow Keyan's care outside of the rehab hospital. He asked permission to come in. When he entered the room, he quietly walked over to Keyan's bedside and stood there—looking at her and taking it all in. Keyan was in the throes of fever, pain, fatigue, and confusion. She was sleeping restlessly. There was great concern evident in his eyes. After standing near Keyan and gently rubbing her shoulder for a short time, he turned and asked if he could sit down on the couch next to me.

He sat and did not say anything for a little while. I could tell his heart was heavy. When he finally spoke, his words were ones I will never forget. He said, "Do you realize that if things don't somehow change for Keyan, she will die from one of these infections?"

While those are words no parent ever wants to hear, I felt an immediate sense of relief upon hearing them. Intuitively, I felt Keyan's health was declining and her life was at risk. But no doctor ever broached the subject with us. When we tried to discuss Keyan's prognosis it was always, "She just needs to grow and get stronger. Give her some more time." We heard this over and over again. Despite what the doctors were saying, we felt we were living a different reality—the reality that her body was failing her.

Confronting your child's mortality is not easy. However, as we watched Keyan get sicker and sicker with each life-threatening infection, we knew the possibility of losing her was real, despite the fact no one on Keyan's care team wanted to talk about it. I believe her doctors were so invested in her care and wanted so badly for her to thrive that they did not want to face the harsh reality of Keyan's decline.

Her physiatrist, on the other hand, took the risk of upsetting me and asked the tough questions. The day he came to see Keyan in the hospital he brought a brochure from the Pediatric Early Care team with hospice. He asked if we wanted him to make a referral. He also explained what palliative care was and how the hospice team could help us make decisions that would ensure Keyan's quality of life was the top priority.

I softly cried as we talked through some of the options. I felt a tremendous weight lift from my shoulders. Finally, someone put words to my fears and gave me and my husband the freedom to explore what our hearts desired for Keyan.

Having Keyan on hospice means we minimize the investigative medical care and focus on comfort care. We forgo sleep studies, routine bronchoscopies, and EEGs because the information gathered will not change her course of care. When doctors push for a test or want to add another treatment to Keyan's routine care, we let them know we are working with the Early Care hospice team. Once they understand what our focus is, they generally yield to our wishes. Informing Keyan's doctors that we are making palliative care decisions gives us a louder voice and a bigger say in her health care decisions.

We also allow Keyan to experience life despite the risks. She gets in the swimming pool, goes to camp, and tastes ice cream. It means something different to every family, but for us, being part of the Early Care hospice team has given us a great resource to make sure that we are not making selfish decisions for Keyan. It opened the door for conversations with other doctors and nurses who care for her with the hope they will understand and accept our intentions—to live with no regrets.

We will be forever indebted to the physiatrist for engaging in the difficult conversation that no one else could. He helped us begin the journey of focusing on Keyan's quality of life. Had we lost Keyan during those first 6 years, we would have a lot of regrets to confront. Now, when or if that day comes, I believe we can say with confidence that we did everything we could to make every day we have with Keyan the best day possible.

Parent Commentary

Parents of medically complex children recognize the toll that repeated illnesses and hospitalizations have on their fragile child. We are educated about our child's disease and understand that our child lives with a life-limiting condition. We know in our hearts when it is time to talk about palliative care or end-of-life decisions. However, someone has to initiate these difficult discussions.

Being told that your child's disease or condition has progressed to the point that they might die is certainly difficult to hear. I can only imagine how difficult it is for a physician to convey this information. Physicians may fear that talking about the child dying risks destroying hope or losing the parent's trust. Parents may fear that talking about their child dying feels like they are giving up. Yet, it is the physicians who have the most knowledge when it comes to disease progression, and they have access to information about the resources available to support the child and family. By braving the difficult conversation with Keyan's mom, the physiatrist did not take away hope or lose her trust. He empowered Keyan's parents to take an active role in her treatment plan going forward and gave them the confidence to accept or decline treatments based on what they thought was best for Keyan. He gave them the resources (Early Care Hospice Team) and the words (palliative care) they needed to convey to other physicians when challenged or questioned for the decisions they were making for their daughter.

Parents do not want to be protected from the truth of their child's disease or decline. They need to know the truth and they want information to help them prepare and plan. Advance care planning discussions should be ongoing, depending on the readiness of the family. Keyan's parents were ready to engage in the discussion.

By compassionately initiating a conversation, physicians open the lines of communication and begin the difficult but necessary discussion with parents about advance care planning and the decisions they will ultimately face as their child's health declines.

Physician Commentary

I empathize with Keyan's mom and salute this physician for beginning the difficult conversation described. In my experience, it is more often than not the physicians who see a dark tunnel ahead for a patient and do not find parents on the same page. But this story illustrates the situation can go both ways. Parents may fear their child will not recover from another setback while the physicians soldier on, fighting each battle as if it would mean winning the whole war. This seems to be the situation here. Finding that tipping point when families and physicians are perfectly aligned in these situations can take time to achieve. Often, it takes a brave physician (as in this case) or an even braver parent to speak up and say: "My child might not survive this setback."

A larger message is illustrated here: the modern role of palliative care. Although we often lump "hospice" and "palliative care" together, they are definitely not the same thing. With the disclaimer that I am not a palliative care physician, typically hospice refers to true end-of-life care, where the patient has a short predicted life expectancy and all care is directed toward comfort only. Palliative care, on the other hand, represents a dynamic range of support for patients and families that does not presume a particular endpoint, but rather endeavors to balance the benefits and burdens intended to prolong a meaningful quality of life for the child. The palliative care team, including physicians, nurses, advanced practice providers (most commonly nurse practitioners), social workers, psychologists, and others, has the resources and the time to explore patients' and parents' goals and values, and can help navigate the often complex teams of consultants who, as well intended as they may be, are often focused on the organ system they are trained to manage. The palliative care physician and multidisciplinary team helps families see the bigger picture. In addition, they are uniquely attuned to management of chronic pain and discomfort, thus helping to ensure that whatever path is chosen is managed with the child's comfort foremost in mind. This modern brand of pediatric palliative care is, as with most new fields, insufficiently staffed in all but the most robust Children's Hospitals. If your home institution does not yet offer this service, it is all the more important to identify a champion physician who can help you navigate the big picture, based on the child's best interests.

A Roadmap

25

5-year-old boy with a complex history.

Complex history. Words that roll off our tongues with ease and without a second thought. But what do we mean when we say these words as health care providers? We speak to each other, sometimes unaware of our audience, grouping our patients into medical jargon terms. We fail to remember that each child is unique. We forget that terms like this can hinder our relationships with our patients and their parents. We unknowingly put a strain on our ability to connect with them, which is already a challenge in the Pediatric Intensive Care Unit. It is our communication and interactions with these parents and patients that shape their perception of us as providers in the PICU. One encounter I recall so vividly.

It was in the middle of winter; one of the busiest and most hectic seasons in any pediatric ICU. When I finally get a chance to look out the window, there is snow falling. I think to myself, "Wow, when did that start?" I catch a glimpse of the people walking on the streets all bundled up in their winter garments, braving the below-freezing temperatures. Two seconds of staring outside before I am snapped back into the chaos of the unit by my pager. It reads: "Bed 10's mom is here. She missed rounds and would like an update." I call the nurse back.

I'll stop by in a few minutes, is that okay?

That's fine, but she is frustrated.

Did something happen?

No, but she was not here on rounds and no one has been by all day.

This mom had been here for quite some time with her son, Ivan. On rounds earlier in the week, there had been an incident with one of the other physicians in the ICU where she became upset and angry with that day's plan for her son. She was

© Springer Nature Switzerland AG 2021
A. F. Schrooten, B. P. Markovitz, *Shared Struggles*,
https://doi.org/10.1007/978-3-030-68020-6_25

frustrated that her son was not making progress. She was distressed over the words that were used to describe her son on rounds. She was upset that the team was not taking her opinions and thoughts about what was best for her son into consideration.

After receiving the page, my initial reaction is frustration. This is another task added to my list. I am already responsible for answering three pagers, giving a lecture to the residents this afternoon, and caring for the 23 other patients in the ICU. I have a preconceived notion that this will not be an easy conversation.

Then I feel exhaustion. I have already worked 70 hours this week. I am two shifts away from 2 days off, and I most definitely need that break that seems so close, yet so far away. After these initial feelings, I feel guilt. Guilt from having these feelings of exhaustion. Guilt because this is someone's son who is in the ICU. Guilt that I put my feelings before that of my patient.

Ivan was born prematurely and because of this, he has complex medical needs. He requires oxygen around the clock for his chronic lung disease, plus two times a day breathing treatments. He had a shunt placed to drain the excess fluid on his brain and, in his short 5 years of life, he has had multiple shunt revision surgeries due to shunt-related complications. He has multiple seizures a day that require him to take his medications six times a day. If he misses a dose, he is likely to be hospitalized. He is unable to walk and spends most of his time in his wheelchair or bed. He also has significant contractures to his body that have resulted in multiple fractures and hip dislocations. Ivan is seen by a team devoted entirely to managing children with medical needs similar to his. They follow him during his healthy periods with clinic visits and also while he is sick in the hospital as consultants. They have developed a relationship with the family and serve as Ivan's primary care team. Although his lungs are rarely sick and he does not require a tracheostomy or home ventilator, Ivan is no stranger to the ICU.

This admission, however, was different. Ivan was not in the ICU for seizures or EEG monitoring, which were his normal reasons for admission. This time, it was pneumonia. A respiratory illness on top of his already frail health. He escalated quickly from high flow nasal cannula to a BiPAP machine to intubation and a ventilator. By the time I met Ivan, he had been intubated for about a week and a half. He was not making huge strides and many days seemed to be one step forward, two steps back. We were escalating his respiratory treatments and ventilator settings, rather than weaning them. The virus he was infected with was taking its toll on his struggling lungs.

This admission was confusing for Ivan's mother. He had not been this sick in quite some time. His longest ICU admission was when he was born. She was not familiar with every alarm that went off. She could not quite comprehend why he was not improving. She was frustrated that he was getting worse every day and she felt that we were not doing anything to help him.

I arrive at Ivan's room a short 5 minutes after my pager snapped me out of my winter wonderland daydream. I immediately notice the four letters spelling out his name with Disney character prints taped to the sliding glass door which leads to his room. There are also pictures of him healthier and in his wheelchair. In one particular picture, he is smiling the biggest, brightest smile with Mickey Mouse ears on his head and Cinderella's castle in the background. When I enter the room, that is not the little boy I see in the bed. He is thinner and he has edema around his eyes. He has a breathing tube in place of his smile and every contracture in his body seems much more apparent than in those pictures. He does not look like the smiling boy at Disney World, and I immediately understand his mother's heartbreak and frustration.

Ivan's mom is in the back of the room, her head shaking in her hands as she talks to Ivan's father on speakerphone. I reintroduce myself to her, as we had met earlier in the week. She hangs up the phone. I ask her if now is a good time to talk and update her on her son's care. She interrupts me before I can start, "Why is he not getting better? I don't understand." I explain to her in the best way I can, "Every child and their recovery is different. The amount of time it could take for his lungs to heal can be days to weeks, we can't be sure. What we can be sure of is that he is showing us that he still needs more time." As she looks at me, I can see every emotion on her face. Exhaustion. Frustration. Fear. Anguish. Hopelessness. She asks, "Am I ever going to have my son back?"

It was at this point I realize that although her son has complex needs, she has never experienced this before. In the ICU, this is something we see every day. But for her, this is new and this is scary. This is unfamiliar territory and she needs a road map. All this mother wants is her smiling boy back. So, despite the chaos in the ICU and the continued tasks building up on my to-do list, this is my priority. What this mother needs at this time is clear communication from a provider. She also needs hope. She needs me to tell her that she will get her smiling boy back. I take a moment to sit in the chair next to her. I put my pagers and phones on "Do Not Disturb." All my focus is on her and her son.

I tell her that Ivan's lungs are sick and I describe in detail how the virus which made him ill has caused an inflammation cascade in his lungs. I draw pictures of his lungs so she can better understand. I explain that he has acquired a bacterial infection and we must tailor our antibiotic regimen to the specific bacteria that is causing his pneumonia. I walk her through his X-Rays and CT scans, describing what I am seeing and how it affects him. I list every single medication that is new and tell her why it is part of his regimen. I explain that every time we make a change it is to help Ivan, not hurt him. I let her know that herself, nurses, therapists, and doctors, including myself, all share a common interest: the best possible outcome for Ivan. I tell her I am working every day to make his comfort our priority. Then I pause. I look at her. She is engaged and following along, listening to every word intently. She is taking notes in her notebook so she can share the information with her husband. Although I am concerned that this is the first time she has heard some of these things, I am also relieved as the frustration and anguish that once appeared on her face have now been replaced with hope and energy. I ask her, "What is most important to you?" She replies, "Small progress every day." I tell her, "And that is our goal."

I leave the room and my initial feelings of frustration, exhaustion, and guilt are replaced with relief and fulfillment. I am so glad I took 15 minutes away from the chaos of the unit to bring some sense of hope to the mother of my patient, because she is hurting too. The unit survived for the few minutes I was away, while this mother's hope was hanging on by a thread.

For the next 2 days, I continue to check in with Ivan and his mother. We consider the smallest moves forward as accomplishments and the small progress we have agreed upon as a common goal. As I check-in for one last time, a note has been left for me with a small memento, an angel with a stethoscope. The note reads:

> .... It has been very hard for us as parents to be here and for our son to have a doctor like you on his team who continues to work so hard and heartedly for his best interest is very much appreciated.

Tears well in my eyes. Clear communication. Fifteen minutes away from the chaos. Treating their son as the unique and special child he is.

This encounter left an imprint on my heart and a lesson I will carry with me for the rest of my career. The angel sits on my bookshelf as a reminder that taking time with my patient's family often gives them exactly what they need: communication and hope.

Parent Commentary

For the parent of a medically complex child who has been admitted to the hospital, there is nothing more maddening than the hours upon hours spent sitting in your child's hospital room. It can feel incredibly frustrating when the health care team of doctors, nurses, respiratory therapists, and techs are in and out of your child's room, all doing their jobs but sharing little information. There may be a plan of care in place (and there very likely is), but if the plan is not communicated to us, we cannot help but feel like nothing is being done to move our child toward improvement and discharge. The hours of waiting in silence and uncertainty give rise to feelings of fear and frustration. Communication is everything.

Admittedly, experienced parents of medically complex children can be high maintenance. We have acquired a great amount of knowledge throughout the years of caring for our child. We ask a lot of questions, we have a lot of opinions, and we are often impatient. We spend a great amount of energy trying to keep our child "healthy"—meaning, we do everything in our power to keep our child out of the hospital. We can manage most of our child's intense medical needs outside of the hospital due to advancements in medical technology that can be used in the home. Our ability to manage our child's complex care at home gives us a sense of control over an otherwise unimaginable way of life. We establish our new normal, find our comfort zone, and ride it out for as long as we can. This belief that we are in control may be illusory, but it is what keeps us sane. When our child ends up in the hospital, much of our frustration stems from a loss of control. We do not like when unknown issues and illnesses come up and we are unable to manage our child on our own at home. This loss of control both scares us and frustrates us. I think it is also fair to say that our threshold for tolerating being knocked out of our comfort zone and losing our sense of control diminishes exponentially over the years. Honestly, we live in a state of perpetual exhaustion trying to maintain control of our child's health, which can take a turn for the worse very quickly. Being in the hospital is the pinnacle of being out of control, and it only piles on to our exhaustion.

If I can suggest anything, it is to communicate with us often, even more so than you might with the parent who will likely only see the inside of the PICU once in their child's lifetime. Do not assume that because we are knowledgeable parents that we do not need the extra attention or hand holding. On the contrary, we need more of it. We need to regain some sense of control, and the physician caring for our child is the one person who can give that back to us by communicating with us often and without us having to ask. Like Ivan's mom, we need and notice the physician who takes the time to sit with us, listens to our concerns, communicates what is going on now, and what the plan is going forward. Your time and attention helps ease the frustration of being in the hospital and preserves our strength—strength we will need after we leave the hospital and return home to the ongoing and often overwhelming demands of caring for our child.

Physician Commentary

Although I should have learned this lesson years ago (maybe I did and have suppressed it), but reading this story was eye opening to me. I too tend to think of the medically sophisticated parents of these complex children as super strong and resilient. I felt they responded to facts, plain and simple. Some of these parents basically are running a home ICU; surely, they are not fazed by being back in a "real" one. How wrong that assumption is on my part.

Just as physicians should tailor their care and communication to each child and family based on the situation and their needs, the families of these children deserve this level of support at least as much. To realize that such "controlling" personalities are knocked off their tracks as much if not more than "normal" parents by having a child in the ICU is a truly illuminating lesson that physicians need to learn.

At least in the PICU, sometimes physicians may, perhaps consciously, or perhaps subconsciously, avoid regular detailed conversations with these parents, fearing they will get drawn into a lengthy meeting that they can ill afford to attend, given all the demands of a busy ICU. However, as occurred in this story, physicians need not harbor this fear indiscriminately. More frequent short conversations may accomplish the objective of improved communication (and providing hope) rather than avoiding them. Because as we have heard, the longer these families go without detailed updates the more frustrated they (rightly) become, and then the time you meet with them (finally) is guaranteed to be a longer and more stressful meeting!

Teamwork

26

My sweet, happy, and stubborn 11-year-old daughter, Keturah, was born with a host of medical complications. None of which define her, but all of which significantly impact her day-to-day life. Keturah was born with bilateral vocal cord paralysis, intestinal malrotation, and a structural defect of her cerebellum known as Chiari I malformation. Keturah also has a condition called congenital central hypoventilation syndrome (CCHS)—a rare disorder which affects her respiratory control and autonomous nervous system regulation. Because of CCHS, Keturah's brain does not tell her body to breathe when she is sleeping. As a result, she has to be connected to a ventilator at night and any time she falls asleep. Keturah has a tracheostomy (trach) to give her a stable airway to support her life-long ventilation needs.

When she was 4 months old, Keturah was diagnosed with a platelet aggregation defect. Her bleeding dysfunction causes bruising and, more significantly, hemoptysis—coughing up blood. When Keturah has a respiratory infection, the hemoptysis can be severe enough to cause hemorrhaging. Blood will literally pour from her trach faster than we can suction it. As a parent, it is horrifying to watch your child cough up massive amounts of blood.

Keturah is not seen on a regular basis in the hematology clinic at our Children's Hospital for her platelet disorder. Because her bleeding is unpredictable and random, I have always been told by the hematology team that Keturah only needs to see them on an as-needed basis when she is bleeding. Yet, when Keturah is bleeding and I call for an appointment, they do not want to see her in clinic. They prefer we manage her at home with medication. As a result, I have never developed as solid a relationship with the hematologist as I have with Keturah's other specialists.

A couple of weeks before a scheduled routine bronchoscopy (bronch) and sleep study, Keturah was sick with a respiratory infection. As is usually the case when she gets a respiratory infection, she started bleeding when she coughed. I called the pulmonologist and asked for an antibiotic. I also called the hematologist for a refill on one of Keturah's bleeding prescriptions and made them aware of her bleeding.

After finishing a 5-day course of several different medications to try and control her bleeding, Keturah's bleeding was still severe. I called the hematologist's office to ask if they wanted to see her in clinic or if they wanted her to get a platelet transfusion to stop the bleeding. The on-call doctor told me to bring her to the emergency department of our Children's Hospital.

The hematologist called ahead so when we arrived at the emergency department we skipped triage and went straight back to a room. The pulmonologist came to see Keturah and discussed possibly scoping her airway in the emergency department to see if he could locate the source of her bleeding. Given that she had a respiratory infection, we agreed it was probably a tear in her mucosal lining from coughing. Because she already completed multiple courses of medications to stop the bleeding, we decided to wait and see what the hematologist thought before proceeding with a bronch.

Four hours after our arrival, the nurse informed me that the hematologist looked at her labs in the computer and called to tell them her platelets looked fine. They did not want to do a platelet transfusion. An hour later, the resident told me she spoke with the hematologist over the phone and that they had two options for Keturah: be admitted to Pediatric Intensive Care Unit (PICU) for observation and to try to move up her scheduled bronch or go home and do another course of medication.

I explained that if they did not want to give her platelets, I was not going to expose her to other illnesses by being in the hospital. I also did not want her to have her bronch when she was sick. We opted to go home and start another course of medication. I asked the resident if we were supposed to give the entire 5-day course again. She said that she did not know and that I would have to call the hematology clinic. At no point during our time in the emergency department did the hematologist come to see Keturah even though we were there at his instruction.

When we got home, I called the pharmacy for a refill of the medication. I was told they needed to contact the hematologist to approve another refill. The pharmacy called back to let me know that the hematologist's office would not refill the prescription because Keturah had not been seen in clinic in over a year. I could not believe what I was hearing. We just left the emergency department where the hematologist told us to go. Yet, he did not come to see Keturah and now his office was refusing to refill her medication. I called the hematology nurse practitioner directly and, thankfully, she called in the prescription.

After completing another 5-day course of medication and continued antibiotics, Keturah's bleeding finally stopped, just in time for her scheduled bronch and sleep study. Coordinating the bronch and sleep study together is difficult and must be done months in advance. The morning of the procedures, the pulmonary nurse called to tell me the doctor scheduled to perform the bronch was canceling until the hematologist gave Keturah clearance because it had been longer than a year since she had seen the hematologist. I asked who canceled. It was a new pulmonologist we had never seen or spoken with.

I explained that we had just been in the emergency department the previous week and the hematologist cleared Keturah to come home; that an option had been to move her bronch up to last week when she was still bleeding; that she had not had fevers in over a week or any bleeding in days; and that she had completed a 14-day course of antibiotics. I asked the nurse to please ask the new pulmonologist to call the pulmonologist who saw Keturah in the emergency department because he knew Keturah and her history well. The doctor refused to make the call. I explained that every time Keturah bleeds, I call the hematology nurse practitioner and request a clinic appointment and I am always told it is not necessary. The doctor still refused to make any calls and canceled the bronch.

I was angry. We had the procedures scheduled months in advance. We chose to do it over spring break to eliminate the amount of time Keturah would miss school. We sacrificed a portion of our family time and her vacation time—days that are supposed to be fun as a child—to be in the hospital for 2 days. We would not be able to reschedule the combination of bronch and sleep study for at least another 4 months.

The canceling of the bronch had a tremendous domino effect. We still moved forward with the overnight sleep study and had to make the hour drive to the hospital. The next week, I had to make the drive again to take Keturah to see the hematologist so he could clear her for the bronch. The rescheduling of the bronch required me to rearrange my work schedule once again and caused Keturah to miss more school. Keturah had to go to the hospital the afternoon before the rescheduled bronch to the outpatient infusion center to get a platelet transfusion. Our one trip to the hospital multiplied into four trips. Keturah's one night of anxiety and stress over getting an IV and having to go under anesthesia became three times the anxiety for her. The 2 days I was prepared to be away from my family became 5 days.

More significantly, everything was now out of order. Keturah's bronch was supposed to come before her sleep study. If the pulmonologist upsizes her trach during the bronch, the settings on her ventilator can be properly adjusted during the sleep study. She had the sleep study with her current trach size. If it is determined she needs a larger trach after the bronch, her ventilator settings will no longer be calibrated based on her then current information.

Teamwork. It is necessary to optimally manage a medically complex child's care. This particular time, it failed miserably. Why? Because the hematologist repeatedly denied my requests for a clinic visit to discuss a treatment plan for the future based on Keturah's current symptoms; because the hematologist did not take the time to see Keturah in the emergency department when he requested she go there; because the pulmonologist refused to call another doctor who is part of their own specialty team to discuss my child with the doctor who knew her and her history; because that same pulmonologist would not call the hematologist to touch base about Keturah.

What terrifies me more than having a child who is medically complex and fragile is having a medical team of specialists who do not communicate with each other. That is when accidents happen. That is when quality of life for patients and families suffer. Unnecessary stress is placed on everyone involved. It takes a long time to gain trust with a medical team and actually feel like the cogs are all meshing together like a well-oiled machine. It only takes one bad experience to break it all down and take all of that trust away and create barriers between the doctors and their patient's caregivers.

Parent Commentary

Our children with multiple, chronic health conditions require ongoing care from as many as ten or more pediatric specialists. This necessarily requires extraordinary levels of collaboration and coordination among and between our child's team of specialists. Our children need coordination of care in the scheduling of appointments, procedures under anesthesia, goals of care, and sharing of information. The cornerstone in managing the chronic and acute needs of our children is communication: communication with the parent and communication and sharing of information with other members of our child's care team. While parents assume much of the responsibility for coordinating care and communication, we cannot carry this burden alone. We need cooperation from every member of our child's care team—from the schedulers, the office staff, and the physicians.

In this story, there was an unfortunate lack of communication and coordination of care between two subspecialties and between subspecialists in the same department, which resulted in additional anxiety and stress for Keturah and her mother. When physicians are unaware of or insensitive to the needs of their patient, the consequences can be far reaching and extend beyond the patient to the parents and the family as a whole. While it may go without saying, patients and parents have lives outside of the microcosm of the clinic and hospital. Parents have job responsibilities and other children to care for. Patients have school and other activities they participate in. A tremendous amount of time and scheduling is involved to coordinate work schedules, school schedules, extracurricular activities, and family vacations around routine clinic visits and procedures. When you add in an acute and urgent medical issue for our child, plans can unravel quickly. Yet we become proficient at finding a way to keep plans on track despite the inevitable interruptions that come with having a medically complex child.

Here, Keturah's bleeding that resulted from a respiratory infection was an acute but known issue. Her mother knew who to call and what was needed to manage the bleeding and avoid the derailment of the meticulously scheduled bronchoscopy and sleep study. It was not Keturah's acute issue that threw the plans off track, it was the failure of Keturah's doctors to talk with each other.

Physicians who care for children with complex medical conditions need to appreciate that they are one member of a multidisciplinary team of subspecialists who care for our child, and it is essential that each physician on the team be willing to take the extra time to communicate and share information with other physicians on the team. It is also important to understand and appreciate the tremendous amount of time and energy required of parents to manage their child's complex medical needs while also managing jobs, households, and the needs of their other children. Something as simple as making a phone call to another physician on your patient's care team can have an impact far greater than you may ever realize.

Physician Commentary

This is a truly unfortunate—and preventable—situation that Keturah and her family experienced. Sadly, this is not unusual. When children are in the ICU, the ICU physician and the ICU team are the "ringleader" and are able (not always successfully[1]) to coordinate the multispecialty care these children require. But there is rarely a "conductor" to coordinate their care once they are home. In some cases, this leadership falls on the patient's primary pediatrician, but this is rare. Sometimes one subspecialist, perhaps the pulmonary medicine doctor in the case of children needing chronic respiratory support, takes on this role. But there is no "standard of care" in these situations.

At my hospital and at more and more Children's Hospitals, a new service has emerged for just this purpose: the Complex Care Team. This is a multidisciplinary team, usually composed of physicians, advance practice providers (nurse practitioners, physician assistants), social workers, and others whose job is to coordinate the care of the complex children, both during and after their hospitalization. They provide the continuity and communication bridge that is so vital and span the spectrum from inpatient to outpatient as well. These teams should be able to provide much needed improvement in communication between families and subspecialists, communication that can not only limit unnecessary care and hardship—as in the case described here—but can be a matter of life and death as well.

---

[1] Suboptimal communication between subspecialty services in the ICU, despite everyone's best efforts, has stubbornly remained a consistent source of family dissatisfaction.

Relearning to Listen

27

As a pediatric intensivist, I spend my days making time-sensitive decisions to provide life-saving interventions to children. After initiation of each intervention, I re-evaluate the child's condition to determine their response and adjust my therapies accordingly. I chose the pediatric critical care specialty because I craved this type of continuity—the instant gratification related to my patient care decisions. The field of pediatric critical care is now transitioning from caring predominantly for patients with acute critical illness and short Pediatric Intensive Care Unit (PICU) stays to a large proportion of children with chronic critical illness and prolonged PICU stays. Our group recognized the need for "PICU continuity physicians" to support patients and families as they navigate the weeks, and sometimes months, of critical care interventions from a revolving door of bedside providers. In this role as a continuity physician, I relearned to listen to my patients' and their families' needs.

I first met Jacob when he was 5 months old, having spent his entire life in the intensive care unit. He had multiple prenatally diagnosed congenital anomalies and was delivered prematurely via urgent c-section for fetal distress. He was intubated shortly after birth due to respiratory failure and was transferred to the local Children's Hospital for better management of his congenital anomalies. Jacob spent his first 4 months of life in the Neonatal Intensive Care Unit where he underwent tracheostomy placement for micrognathia, a small jaw, and need for long-term ventilator support and continued management of his other medical conditions, which included congenital hypothyroidism, seizure disorder, poor intestinal motility, low muscle tone, and developmental delay. Given his age and need for long-term critical care, he was transferred to the Pediatric Intensive Care Unit.

I arranged a family care conference at the end of my week of service to update Jacob's mother on his clinical status and discuss his general goals of care. During that week, he developed a severe systemic bacterial infection, requiring antibiotics and medications to support his blood pressure, increased settings on the ventilator, and additional medications to control his increased seizures. I knew it would not be an easy conversation with his mother. She sat calmly in the room with the multidisciplinary providers and interpreter and listened to our updates with a facial

© Springer Nature Switzerland AG 2021   135
A. F. Schrooten, B. P. Markovitz, *Shared Struggles*,
https://doi.org/10.1007/978-3-030-68020-6_27

expression showing both worry and strength simultaneously. When I asked her to share her concerns, I noted a change in her expression. She clearly articulated concerns about inadequate communication regarding Jacob's clinical status on a daily basis. She wanted to know all the details of his care, which our team mistakenly assumed would not be of interest or important to her. With her determined eyes full of strength, she made it clear that she would be Jacob's best advocate. At the same time, I knew I would become Jacob's PICU continuity physician.

After that conference, we transitioned to providing detailed daily updates with an interpreter. I checked in with Jacob's mother regularly, and I could see the sense of relief on her face. For her, knowledge about the details of her son's care was power. How could she ever take care of her son if she did not understand all he had been through? Over time, her need for my involvement decreased and Jacob ultimately improved enough to transfer out of the PICU when he was 6 months old. Unfortunately, his initial stay on the inpatient ward was short—only 10 days. He bounced back and forth between the PICU and the inpatient ward two more times over the course of a month. On his third PICU readmission, I knew I needed to increase my involvement.

At the time, Jacob was suffering from feeding intolerance that was so severe that his distended abdomen made ventilation difficult, resulting in his inability to successfully transition to a home ventilator. His oxygen levels would intermittently drop despite ventilator adjustments and frequent pausing of his enteral formula. His prognosis appeared grim. We scheduled a multidisciplinary care conference with his parents to talk about challenges with his management and his lack of improvement.

I conveyed that I was not sure whether we could ever get Jacob home. Upon hearing my concerns, Jacob's mother, sitting next to her husband and holding his hand, looked me straight in the eye and said, "We don't have hope that Jacob will ever leave the hospital."

The power of her words smacked me in the face. I had been talking with staff for weeks about Jacob. Some questioned whether his mother truly understood the severity of his illness. Some questioned our medical decision-making that included ordering aggressive workups for changes in his clinical status and initiating new life-sustaining therapies, even if they may be painful. But I knew she understood. With a mother's love, she told me many times that every day with Jacob was a gift to her and her family. Yet now, in the face of multiple complications, she thought we had reached a turning point. It was time to change course.

While keeping Jacob's comfort in the forefront, we developed a plan to restart enteral feeds at a very low rate and increase the volume in the slowest possible manner to evaluate the impact on his breathing. This was his test—he needed to prove that he could tolerate enteral formula so we could stop his intravenous nutrition that comes with a high risk of life-threatening infection. I checked in regularly at the bedside with his mother to see how he was doing with this advance. When I entered his room, I could always tell how he was doing by her facial expression, so her verbal response to my questions merely confirmed what I already knew. Day by day, he tolerated the feeding advance and reached his daily caloric goal just before his first birthday.

To celebrate Jacob's birthday, his parents arranged a party for him and for the staff. "Bring your appetite," his father instructed me a few days before the party. The event was unforgettable. There sat Jacob in his chair, wearing a suit and a crown, surrounded by family and the staff who had cared for him since birth. When some of us suggested we might not have room for dessert after the homemade meal, his father insisted, "Today is not for dieting. It is for celebrating." Just before they brought out his smash cake, they gave a little speech. "This party is for Jacob, but it is also for you. We want to thank you because we didn't know if we would ever see this day. We are so thankful for all the hard work you have done to help Jacob make it to this day. Thank you."

I was overwhelmed with emotion. There they stood, a family that had struggled through an entire year of their son's critical illness. And they thanked us. Despite all the painful procedures, lab draws, early morning disruptions to examine Jacob, and communication challenges, they were grateful. It was just like they told me months ago—every day with Jacob was a gift.

Jacob eventually improved enough to leave the PICU—this time for good. When he was 17 months old, Jacob was discharged home from the hospital. I went to visit him the day of his discharge, expecting to see nothing but joy on his mother's face. Joy was definitely there, but there was also a bit of trepidation. She expressed concerns about being able to take care of him—giving all the medications on time and all other aspects of his care. I reassured her that she was ready. She had been at his bedside for 17 months and knows his needs better than anyone. I had no doubt she would be able to provide excellent care for him. After a lovely conversation, she thanked me again, reiterating how appreciative their family was for the care he received and mentioning that she didn't think this day would ever come. I felt the same way.

When I first started caring for Jacob, I shared many of the concerns of my colleagues related to ongoing aggressive therapies for Jacob. I doubted whether those interventions were worth the suffering. I worried that Jacob would spend his entire life in our hospital despite our best efforts. I feared that his family did not fully understand the medical complexity and would end up regretting those painful procedures in the future. By spending extra time with Jacob and his family and by listening to their thoughts and fears, I began to understand their doubts, worries, and fears. At the same time, I also started to appreciate their hope and resilience. Of course, they did not want their precious child to suffer—but they did want as much time with him as possible. Each day with him was a gift. After all those months in the hospital, I was humbled by how much their gratitude continued to flow. But no matter how grateful they are to us, I must be more grateful to them.

The time spent with Jacob and his family, listening to their thoughts and fears without the typical PICU time constraints and guiding them through tough decision-making, made me a better physician. They taught me the importance of taking extra time to truly listen. Only when you truly listen can physicians begin to understand a family's perspective and then offer guidance and support that aligns with their goals. Jacob reshaped my approach to pediatric critical care by teaching me to listen. For that, I will forever remain grateful.

Parent Commentary

The last place any parent expects to care for their newborn baby is inside an intensive care unit. Initially, we feel overwhelmed and lost in this new world of medical technology and information. However, for those of us whose child spends months in the intensive care unit, we listen, observe, and eventually acquire some understanding of medical-speak. And just like any parent, we still want to parent our child even if they are living in a foreign environment connected to tubes and wires. We instinctively step into the role of our child's advocate. Some of us may be more vocal than others; however, as the parent in this story makes clear, a quiet personality or language barrier should not be interpreted to mean a parent does not understand or does not want to know what is going on with their child.

When our child's hospital admission is long term, we cannot help but form relationships with the doctors and nurses who care for our child. We are also keenly aware of the ever-present challenges, devastating losses, and incredible care that takes place in an intensive care environment and their impact, not only on the families of the children but also on the medical team. This doctor seemed surprised that Jacob's parents were deeply appreciative of the care they provided for their son, even though it was often difficult to witness. I think many parents who have spent any significant amount of time in an intensive care unit would agree when I say, "we see you." We are not oblivious to the challenging work you do. You are very much appreciated, and while we do not all have the opportunity or means to throw an in-hospital party before discharge, I have no doubt that if you take the opportunity to talk with us and get to know us as this doctor did, you will hear many of the same sentiments shared by Jacob's parents.

I also understand the trepidation Jacob's mother felt going from participating in Jacob's care within the safety of the hospital walls to managing all his care at home without an ICU team on standby. It is scary and I can say from my own experience that words of encouragement from the doctors and nurses who have walked with us through the hard stuff to get to the point of discharge are instrumental in giving us the confidence we need to walk out the doors of the hospital with our child. At the end of the day, we (doctors and parents) have the same goal—to give our child the best chance possible to live the best life possible. We accomplish this through communication, teamwork, and a mutual appreciation of one another.

Physician Commentary

Here is another poignant example of how rewarding it is for patients, families, and physicians when physicians take the time to listen. Really listen. Walk the walk of the parents. Look at the child through their eyes. Then make sure your goals and plans for the child are aligned. Do not make assumptions about the values of your patients and families. Do not impose your values—usually done implicitly not explicitly, so recognition of this is critical—on them. Caring for these medically complex patients can only be successful as a partnership with their parents.

There are several false assumptions about this mother unearthed in this story. That the mother did not understand the severity of the child's condition. That she did not care about daily updates. That she expected to take the child home. There were probably more that were not mentioned. That this physician learned about these misperceptions and altered the dynamic was admirable. We should constantly have our radar on to look for disconnects and correct them as was done here.

This physician is correct in describing the changing demographics of children in the PICU in the United States. The usual model of care for attending physicians in PICUs is to be "on service"—in charge of all or some of the patients in the unit—for a week at a time. This work is usually intense, and it takes a toll on physicians if we work much longer at a stretch. However, this means the primary intensivist for each patient changes weekly, and this is suboptimal for continuity of care of long-stay patients. More PICUs are moving to this model of a "continuity" attending, to provide a consistency of care over time. Usually these physicians do not make the day-to-day or minute-by-minute decisions on these patients but are rather there for "big picture" discussions and to help facilitate dialogue with families as the primary intensivist, similar to a patient's primary cardiologist or neurologist. This is a model of care to be encouraged and spread.

If your child is in the PICU for a long stay, it is worth asking about a program like this. Even if your PICU does not regularly provide a continuity attending, there is no harm in asking about it. You can even ask your favorite attending (almost always the one who listens and communicates with you the best) to play this role for you and your child. It is just important to realize what their role will be, and it is not to micromanage details, but to help coordinate broader issues and decisions.

Words Matter

28

When you have a child with a chronic medical condition, the days can be a blur, but then a single moment is etched in time, frozen forever. For me, that moment was a Monday evening when I was at work helping to facilitate a meeting. I am a high school math teacher and was at work for a Newcomer Parent Night, a meeting to give information to our refugee families about the ins and outs of the American education system to enable them to better support their children. It was close to the end of the meeting and we were having a question and answer time when my phone rang. My phone was on vibrate in case of an emergency, so it buzzed in my pocket. I was surprised to see that it was from my older son, which was highly unusual. I decided to answer, pushing away the worry. I stepped back from the table I was standing near and answered the phone.

My son frantically said "Javad isn't responsive!"

In the background, I heard my ex-husband yell, "He isn't responsive to me. Come on Javad!"

I yelled, "Hang up and call 911 now! I'll call back."

I quickly gathered my things and rushed to my car. I called home while driving furiously down the freeway. I knew that, at best, I was 25 minutes away. I talked to my brother who helplessly gave the play by play as to what was happening as I barked orders about checking Javad's trach, using the Ambu bag, and suctioning—all things we do when he experiences episodes of distress. My mom came on the phone to inform me that the paramedics were there and that they had begun administering CPR. I continued to drive frantically while they continued to work on him thinking that I should have been there. I felt sick and helpless.

I could hear the paramedics talking about taking Javad to the nearest hospital, as was protocol. I knew that the nearest hospital did not have the ability to care for him due to his medical condition. I yelled into the phone that they needed to take him to our Children's Hospital, the hospital where Javad is known and has received all of his care. Negotiations were taking place as my brother advocated for Javad. Finally, the decision was made that he was stable enough to go to Children's.

© Springer Nature Switzerland AG 2021
A. F. Schrooten, B. P. Markovitz, *Shared Struggles*,
https://doi.org/10.1007/978-3-030-68020-6_28

I met the ambulance at the hospital and Javad was assessed in the emergency department and then whisked upstairs to the pediatric ICU (PICU) to begin a cooling protocol due to his cardiac arrest. Over the next few days, Javad was cooled to 33.2 degrees. The room was so cold, beyond what words can even describe. I bundled up in blankets while Javad slept in his cold slumber. He was as close to death as I could imagine, feeling his cold skin and watching his lifeless body. The cooling process continued for 3 days. During this time, they discovered Javad was having seizures. It was then that things began to make more sense. We believed it was a seizure that caused the event, not a respiratory episode as originally thought. A seizure was something we had never experienced or anticipated.

Javad was 13 years old at the time of the event. He was living with a diagnosis of myotubular myopathy, a rare neuromuscular disease that caused overall muscle weakness. He had been doing incredibly well. He was stronger than most affected individuals his age, maintaining movement in his arms and trunk. He was able to use his iPad for speech, watching movies, and playing video games. He attended school and had friends.

In the blink of an eye, life changed dramatically. I had no idea what the future held. All I knew was that my son was now nearly frozen, asleep, and unable to move at all. The waiting game had begun. Javad continued to have small seizures, but even more concerning to everyone was that he was not showing any signs of waking up. After a week, he was moved out of the PICU and into a room on the floor. He had been cooled and thawed and we were now just waiting for him to heal. He was not moving or waking and the medical team was trying to sort out the next steps. After a few days, I was notified that the team wanted to meet with us in a conference room down the hall.

When doctors want to meet with you alone in a separate room it is never good. I told them that I did not want to go to another room, I wanted to meet in Javad's room. I was assured that the other room would be more comfortable because there was more room for everyone to sit. Despite my protests, the meeting was held in the conference room, as the team requested.

We entered the room—my ex-husband, myself, the nurse manager, a neurologist who I had not met prior to this meeting, and the pediatrician covering the floor. The nurse manager knew our family. She was previously a floor nurse and had cared for Javad when he was younger. She knew our journey, the ups and downs, and the many times Javad had proven medical professionals wrong. I entered the meeting believing that Javad was stable enough that we could begin to put a plan in place to bring him home.

In a flat and clinical tone, the neurologist started the meeting with, "We need to talk about your decision regarding the next steps."

"What do you mean?" I asked.

She said, "Well, he is showing no signs of improvement, no signs of waking up."

Hearing her words, I immediately felt we were being asked to make an end-of-life decision right away, without giving Javad more time to heal. He already depends on a ventilator to support his breathing, but it was inferred that they were asking us if we wanted to discontinue that support.

I could feel my heart rate rise and my stress level increase. I told them, "I think that we are being a little too quick to decide here. Javad has been through a lot. He had a massive seizure, cardiac arrest, three days of cooling, then thawing, then two days of large amounts of medication, and that's just the first week. He is already starting at a deficit because of his underlying disease."

I continued to plead my case, "We can't expect that he will recover the same as a typical child. He is not the same as other children, he started with a big deficit in comparison." But the neurologist persisted and reiterated that we needed to talk about the next steps because Javad was not responding to the medications. Yet, she did not present us with a list of options to consider and no one else in the room said a word.

I began to cry, which is rare for me. I am usually able to handle my emotions. I explained that our plan was to take Javad home and wait for what they might feel was an unreasonable amount of time. Then, after some amount of time that we would determine, we would then look to make decisions, whatever those might be. I stressed that we did not want to rush into making what I believed was an end-of-life decision because it was too early to predict what Javad's future might look like.

I was frustrated because nothing was said about the progress Javad had made or the fact that his seizures were now under control. Neither of the doctors present at the meeting knew Javad. No one asked what Javad's life was like before the event. No one knew what he had already been through and overcome during his lifetime. I needed them to understand that they could not judge Javad's progress on the same scale as other children. He had an underlying neuromuscular disease before he had the seizure. The trauma of the seizure, the cooling protocol, and the massive amounts of drugs he was on would affect him much greater than a typical, otherwise healthy, child. They wanted him to respond like other children and I felt that was unrealistic.

My ex-husband asked if I was ok, because now I was crying quite hard. I told him, "No, I'm not. This isn't the way it's supposed to be." I got up and left the room. I wandered around the halls of the floor trying to calm myself down. After about 30 minutes, I headed back to Javad's room. When I returned to his room, I called our nurse manager. We talked and I told her how disappointed I was with the way the meeting had gone. She expressed that she was surprised with the discussion as it was not what she expected. The doctors in the meeting did not know me or our family, and they definitely did not know Javad. I was angry, hurt, frustrated, and concerned. It was one of the only times I felt defeated when it came to Javad. There had been only a few times in the course of Javad's life that I really wondered what the next steps were. This time, I was filled with tremendous doubt.

I knew another meeting needed to take place. The nurse manager arranged for me to meet with each doctor independently. I met with the floor pediatrician first. He quietly listened while I shared that I did not feel it was right to make sweeping prognostic generalizations about a child who had a major trauma, especially when, as in our case, you are dealing with a child who also had an underlying disease.

I then met with the neurologist. I wanted her to know that this was not our first experience dealing with the unknown. I explained to her that the words she chose gave the impression that she was looking for us to make end-of-life decisions and I did not believe that was how the discussion should have started. She seemed surprised and was apologetic. She explained her statements by saying that she was talking about medication decisions not end-of-life decisions. While I am not convinced that was what she meant at the time, I believe that had she been talking to another family without the experience we had, a life-altering and possibly unwanted decision might have been made.

It has now been 5 years since the "event." The memories are still raw and filled with emotions. Javad still struggles. Once a boy who had some control of his body, it took a year for him to learn how to shake his head "no" again and another 6 months after that to give a small head shake for "yes." Even now, I do not know how much more he will recover, but I do know that if I had been less confident in my son and my own judgment, we might have made a life-ending decision and Javad might not be with us today.

Reflecting on that monumental meeting, I think about the words spoken by the neurologist. I can only imagine how challenging it is for doctors to talk about potential end-of-life decisions with patients' families. If I could go back to that day, I would have handled the meeting very differently from the beginning. I would have stood my ground and insisted that the meeting take place in Javad's room where we were more comfortable. Our comfort should have been a priority. I would have helped the doctors better understand our son. At the onset of the discussion, I wish the doctors had asked about Javad and what he was like before the event. I believe these initial steps would have helped establish a more open and trusting interaction between our family and the medical team.

Words are incredibly powerful, especially when the listener is vulnerable. A doctor's choice and delivery of words makes a difference in how the information is received. If Javad's neurologist was indeed just talking about medication decisions, she should have said that and not phrased her words the way she did. Everything about her opening statement gave the impression that we had very different ideas about the purpose of the meeting and what decisions were being asked of us. It was a meeting that could have changed the course of our lives forever.

Parent Commentary

This story involves a monumental breakdown in communication at a very emotionally charged time. Because of what was not said, assumptions were made by the parent and the physician about the message conveyed. I do not know whether the physician in this story truly meant medication decisions or whether she was unprepared or unwilling to have the difficult end-of-life discussion or whether she chose not to pursue the discussion because of the pushback she was receiving from Javad's mother. Regardless, because of the physician's choice of words, or lack thereof, Javad's mother assumed she was being asked to remove her son from his ventilator—technology he lived with every day of his life. She did not see her son's present condition as one he could not recover from and, therefore, was not ready to take the decision-making discussion any further.

Parents of medically complex children have seen their child become very sick, believing that their child was going to die and, yet, time and time again our child comes through the crisis. How are we or our child's doctors to know if the current illness or event will be the tipping point for our child when they have always come through in the past? The technology that keeps our child alive when they are not acutely ill is also what gives us the hope that they will recover this time and return home, believing that the technology already in place will continue to sustain our child's life. This is the foundation upon which parents stand when their technology-dependent child is critically ill and there is a question of whether support should be discontinued.

The neurologist in this story did not have a history of caring for Javad, and therefore, she did not know him or his baseline. If a physician does not know the child, assumptions can be made about quality of life and what constitutes a good outcome that may not be accurate or fair for that child. Javad was taken to the Children's Hospital because it is where he received care in the past. It is possible that doctors who were part of his regular care team were available and could have been called by the neurologist so she could get a better understanding of Javad's baseline. When caring for a child with an underlying disease that is severely limiting in the best of circumstances, it may be difficult to know how much of what is presented is due to an acute issue and what is baseline, especially when you do not know the child. Listening to the parents who know their child best is essential. In addition, a phone call to one of the doctors on Javad's primary care team might have been helpful to both the neurologist and Javad's family in identifying what needed to be discussed and what decisions needed to be made.

This story also highlights the importance of advance care planning for our children with life-limiting conditions and why discussions surrounding end-of-life decisions should be initiated during a time when our child is stable and not brought up for the first time during a time of crisis. It is important for the physician who knows our child best to initiate advance care planning discussions. Discussions about the "what if" scenarios should take place early on and be continually re-evaluated as our child gets older. We cannot always predict the exact scenario in which we will be asked to consider difficult decisions regarding our child's life. However, the more prepared we are as parents, the better able we will be to be in control of the situation and the decision-making process, and the less chance for miscommunication and misunderstanding on the part of the parent and the physician in a time of crisis.

Physician Commentary

This is a tragic story compounded by suboptimal communications by the physicians, in my opinion. Of course, we do not know what other communications were happening all along after Javad's cardiac arrest before this meeting, but I would never start an important family meeting with what should essentially be the end of the discussion—the decision. Family meetings are a time to share content; how the child is doing, from the perspective of the parents and the physicians. "How do you feel Javad is doing?" "What is your understanding of Javad's condition now?" Based upon answers to questions like these, the physician can then weave in their medical update, so parents and physicians are on the same page in their understanding of the child's current state. It is at this point that prognosis or outlook is brought into the conversation.

I would say that although there are some early predictors of neurologic outcome after cardiac arrest, few carry genuine clarity, and physicians are rarely able to predict with a high degree of certainty what kind and how much recovery a child can make after such an event. (Waking up right after the event is a uniformly good sign!) Although in general we believe children may be more resilient after a period of lack of blood flow to the brain (which causes the neurologic injury from cardiac arrest), it is only relative. So, a range of possible outcomes need to be discussed.

Then it becomes natural for parents and physicians to seek an answer to the question of "What now?" "What are the next steps?" "What are the options and what are the risks and benefits of each?" I would never start a conversation with: "We need to discuss next steps."

Finally, given the range of prognoses, any decision points must incorporate the family's values (and the child's wishes, if they can be known). If in a case like Javad's, the family was told he might never talk again and what his quality of life might look like, some families would accept that as a potential outcome, while others may not. The physician should never impose their own value system upon families. They can only do their best to present the range of possibilities and make their best estimate of the likelihood of these, so the family can make an informed decision about what is best for themselves and their child. A physician should never say: "I know what you are going through," or "if this were my child, I would…." Never.

Trust Their Voice

29

As a pediatrician who specializes in providing primary care to children with medical complexity, a palliative care physician who consults on patients with life-limiting diagnoses, and a hospice physician who is trained to care for children at end of life, I was fortunate to take care of Isabella in all three realms.

Originally, Isabella and I met each other in her eighteenth year of life as I took over as primary care physician. Isabella had been seeing a pediatrician in the community; however, she was starting to have more frequent hospitalizations and specialists' appointments and it was becoming increasingly difficult for her community pediatrician to adequately care coordinate for her medical complexity. As a result, she was referred to our Complex Care Clinic and I became her pediatrician.

Isabella was a beautiful teenager with long, thick, dark brown hair; gentle brown and expressive eyes; and a beautifully full smile. She was originally diagnosed with hydrocephalus requiring multiple shunt revisions and many neurosurgical procedures. She suffered from chronic headaches, and starting at the age of 16, she began to have episodes of dystonia. The muscles of her face and neck would stiffen and cause her head to deviate to the left. These episodes were not predictable and could last hours. As time progressed, the episodes of dystonia involved other muscles in her body. She had many hospitalizations to try to figure out the cause behind these episodes, and over the course of years, she continued a slow decline involving more hospitalizations, more pain, and loss of independent function. Over the course of about 2 years, she lost the ability to walk, feed herself, and sit on her own.

Isabella's mother, who was Spanish speaking only, was a fierce advocate for her daughter and sought many second opinions, but unfortunately was unable to get a more specific diagnosis than "neurodegenerative disorder of unknown etiology." Over the course of the first year taking care of Isabella, it became clear to me that she was very intelligent and wise. She always had a calm demeanor, even speaking as calmly and clearly as she could during a dystonic reaction. Her goals were clear. She wanted to try to get her symptoms controlled as much as possible. My role morphed from pediatrician to palliative care physician and we began to have many conversations about quality of life. We discussed decisions that she might need to

© Springer Nature Switzerland AG 2021
A. F. Schrooten, B. P. Markovitz, *Shared Struggles*,
https://doi.org/10.1007/978-3-030-68020-6_29

make in the future. For example, if her breathing were to worsen, would she want a tracheostomy (artificial airway) and long-term ventilation. We discussed her code status in the event that her heart was to stop or she was to stop breathing on her own. She, along with her mother, had decided that she did not want aggressive resuscitation and that if her breathing were to worsen such that she could no longer breathe on her own, she did not want to be "dependent on machines." While Isabella's muscles were not cooperating with her, she remained cognitively intact and was able to clearly verbalize her goals. Her mother, who was her biggest advocate, was always in support of Isabella's decisions.

After about another year of outpatient visits and a few hospitalizations, Isabella opened up to me that she did not think she was improving with hospitalizations and she did not want to go back to the hospital. It was clear that she and her mother had conversations prior to this appointment. They were both tearing up, as they knew what this statement was suggesting. We had discussed hospice in the past, but until that point, frequent specialist appointments and hospitalizations seemed to be leading to some improvement, if only temporary. However, Isabella was no longer able to see any benefit, and coming to the clinic and to the hospital were increasingly more difficult as she had lost her ability to walk independently. Her dystonic episodes continued daily and were quite painful.

After she was admitted to hospice, Isabella no longer went to her specialists because she felt as if they had nothing more beneficial to offer. I remained involved with her care and, ultimately my role evolved to hospice physician. We were able to have many home visits in which we discussed her symptoms, increased medications to try to combat those symptoms, while trying to make sure she was as awake and alert as possible in order to interact with her family.

While it was clear to me that Isabella was having disease progression, it was difficult to provide a clear prognosis. Her dystonia did seem to be worsening, but she retained the ability to talk and breathe without difficulty. However, Isabella was very clear that she was dying. She would say, "Thank you for taking care of me and my family. Please make sure to take care of them when I am gone." All along Isabella's journey, her major concern was her family. While Isabella suffered significant pain on a daily basis, she wanted to make sure that everyone was going to be okay, especially her mother. Although Isabella had four siblings at home, her mother was by her side 24/7, tirelessly advocating for her.

Isabella seemed to know that the end was coming, certainly more quickly than I was able to predict. She would talk about who she wanted to be at her funeral, what kind of music, what scripture was to be recited, and who was to recite it. Of course as a hospice physician, when a patient is able to make their wishes known, this is celebrated. I felt honored to be part of these conversations, but still was not convinced she was going to die in the next weeks. However, within a few weeks of my last home visit and the one in which she shared the details of her end-of-life wishes, she had an acute worsening of her dystonia. The majority of Isabella's hospice care was provided in the home, but when her symptoms acutely worsened, we admitted her to our inpatient hospice facility for better symptom control and more nursing support. Her dystonia was so severe and medication resistant that we had to use many medications at large quantities. In addition, the inpatient hospice facility was able to provide 24/7 RN care, as well as daily rounding by physicians. While we were giving IV and rectal medications aggressively to try to control her dystonia, she continued to tell me and her family, "I'm going with God. I will be fine. Please take care of each other."

Isabella did eventually stop breathing. I wish I could say that it was peaceful, but her dystonia would not allow that. She was surrounded by all who loved her and she never let that smile leave her face.

Isabella was wise beyond her years and she touched many lives in her short life, including mine. As is known, prognosis is challenging in pediatric patients. Isabella taught me to listen more closely to my patients and families as they often know more than the medical team about their condition and timeline. As a pediatrician who provides hospice care to patients at end of life, I discuss with my patients and their families the signs and symptoms that often present at end of life. However, thanks to Isabella, I now include asking my patients and their families their thoughts on how they feel their disease is progressing. This is a more inclusive approach and often leads to more thoughtful and empathic conversations. Isabella has made me a better person and physician, and for this, I am eternally grateful.

As an update, her mother is now employed at the hospital for which I work. We run into each other every few months. Of course she was struggling soon after Isabella's death, but has since really come toward acceptance, and it shows on her large smile, likely the one that she bestowed on Isabella. We greet each other with a big hug, she updates me on how the family is doing, and we reminisce on how much Isabella is missed and how much her life is celebrated.

Parent Commentary

We often hear that doctors are too pessimistic and unwilling to offer hope when the health of our child with a progressive condition begins to decline. In this story, however, the doctor, while knowledgeable and realistic about her patient's disease progression, was reluctant to predict the end was near even though her patient was telling her otherwise. It is evident that this doctor had a special relationship with her young patient. This story shares an experience that many parents of medically complex children do not get to experience—their child having a voice and an active role in their end-of-life treatment decisions. It is insightful to hear that a child knows when their body is tired, knows that death is near, and wants their parents to know they will be okay. I think for parents whose child is unable to express those feelings when death is near, we sense that our child knows these same things through their nonverbal communication and cues that we have come to know so well. However, as the parent of a child who could not verbally express his feelings at the end of his life, it is powerful and comforting to hear Isabella's words as she prepared her doctor, her mother, and herself for her death.

This story also reinforces the importance of listening to your patient (or their parent). The oft-repeated message from parents about the importance of listening to us because we know our child best applies equally to your young patient who is able to express how they feel and what they need from their doctor. A doctor's knowledge about their patient's disease or condition should always be paired with a patient's (or parent's) intuition.

Isabella displayed incredible grace and compassion for those close to her as she faced her own death. This doctor showed great compassion in honoring Isabella's end-of-life wishes, and in listening to Isabella and learning from her the importance of trusting your patient's voice even it if does not always align with your knowledge and experience.

Physician Commentary

This is a very poignant story of—despite the outcome—hope. There is hope that physicians are learning to listen better to their patients and families. In the medical and lay literature, there has been discussion for years over the concept of "impending doom." Patients can sense changes in themselves that they sometimes cannot even verbalize. I have seen teenagers describe this overwhelming sensation of being about to die, even with normal vital signs. And they are often right. What is unusual to me about Isabella is that she sensed her demise weeks in advance.

However, the most important lesson from this story is not about her death, but about the incredible partnership between herself, her physician, and her mother. The mutual respect and trust they shared is so transparent in this physician's words. The path they forged together could only have occurred the way it did because of the bond they formed over time, together. This is the precise relationship that must occur between patients, families, and physicians of medically complex children to offer them the best outcome. Trust and respect can only come from deep, empathic, and earnest listening.

Knowing Your Family

30

My husband and I often say to each other that Will decided he could not wait any longer to meet his mom and dad, so he arrived 9 weeks early. Though it was a surprise to go into premature labor, I had a strong intuition throughout my pregnancy that my child had unique needs. Looking back, this was one of the wisest lessons Will taught me: never underestimate a mother's intuition. It indeed has been a guiding force throughout our journey.

It was obvious upon birth that Will had significant challenges ahead of him. He struggled to breathe after he was born and was immediately intubated with a breathing tube and placed on a ventilator. He had a weak suck and swallow and had to be fed through a nasal-gastric (NG) tube. The sorting out of what issues were related to prematurity and which ones might be from an overarching medical diagnosis set us on an extended course in the Neonatal Intensive Care Unit (NICU).

We were grateful to be at a world-class medical institution. We knew we were in the right place for Will's medical care, but we did not imagine our first days, weeks, and months as new parents would take place in a hospital, rather than the nursery we prepared in our home. As we approached the 1-month mark, we saw many other families come and go with their babies. We wondered when it would be our turn. Many tests were performed to determine Will's underlying diagnosis. For the first month, every test came back negative and left the medical team guessing. Our partners in this experience were Will's bedside nurses. Our nurses quickly became like family as they witnessed what we were experiencing and showed us ways to care for our son. They helped us create a personal and as comfortable as possible space as we decorated Will's isolette with photos, stuffed animals, and mementos. We tried our best to live life as a new family of three in this semi-public environment, and our team of nurses did their best to support our cherished moments and walk this journey with us.

As Will approached 5 weeks old, a meeting with the medical team was scheduled to discuss the results of his muscle biopsy. It was "THE" meeting in our son's medical journey that was the tipping point for us in so many ways. We entered the

© Springer Nature Switzerland AG 2021
A. F. Schrooten, B. P. Markovitz, *Shared Struggles*,
https://doi.org/10.1007/978-3-030-68020-6_30

meeting with a lot of anxiety and the feeling that the news was not good based on the anxiety the staff displayed toward us.

What surprised us most was the number of people entering the room. It started to feel like Noah's Ark as specialists came in two by two: two neurologists, two neonatologists, two nurses, two respiratory therapists, and others. There were a few familiar faces from the NICU. Many others we did not know at all. A very formal and distant feeling to the conversation was set as the staff took over the boardroom table.

A neurologist we did not know took the lead in relaying information from the biopsy. It was not good news. Will's challenges now had a name—myotubular myopathy or MTM. Although the neurologist spoke clearly, a lot of information was relayed. In almost the same breath as the diagnosis of MTM was given, the decision of whether to continue supportive care of long-term medical technology was placed on the table. The tubes in Will's mouth and nose that kept him breathing and eating were not permanent options. Sooner or later they would have to be replaced surgically. For Will, this involved a tracheostomy to provide a safe airway for long-term ventilation needs and a gastrostomy tube to support long-term nutritional needs. Or, we could choose to remove the current tubes and not replace them with anything. The alternative of withdrawing medical technology would likely result in Will's death.

We listened carefully, but I shutdown in terms of being able to convey my own thoughts. We were deeply saddened by the news. I was also saddened by a complete disconnect we felt from the moment the meeting started. Why would we want a table full of people surrounding us when we received this news? Why were they all there if only one person was conveying the information?

We felt like the objects of "Show & Tell." Show them the data, tell them the choices, and learn from how they react. Although our experience at this teaching hospital was mostly positive, we could not believe every specialty chose our conversation to be a teachable moment. The meeting was postponed for days to get "the team" in place. But where was our team? Where were the people who knew us and with whom we had confided in to this point? This conversation was in stark contrast to the intimate bedside talks we had had with Will's primary care team members in the NICU.

We soon discovered that the grim prognosis they presented for MTM came from a 1970's textbook was not the most up-to-date medical information available. On our own, we found a more recent medical article that discussed how individuals with MTM were surviving longer and having a greater quality of life with medical technology, particularly respiratory support. We subsequently learned that a lead researcher in the world at the time investigating MTM was right there at our hospital. Why was he not called in to participate in the team meeting? By not disclosing the whole picture and all available information, a great divide had begun and it left a big gap in trust moving forward.

In hindsight, our goals for the "big" diagnosis meeting were very different. Our providers would have likely titled this teachable moment "Delivering difficult news of a MTM diagnosis." We wanted the title to be "Telling our family about MTM and how it will affect Will in the context of our unique family." As challenging as it was, that approach would have invited us to begin processing the information as a next step in our journey, starting from where *we* were at, not based on a generic expectation of how a "typical" family might respond.

Every family is unique and high-stake decisions are very personal decisions. Ask us who we would like to have present at the meeting. Inviting the core team who had been at Will's bedside with us and with whom we had had many intimate talks sharing our hopes, visions, and concerns would have gone a long way in minimizing the detachment we felt as critical information was being delivered to us. Had we been asked, we would have requested the involvement of chaplaincy at the meeting. Including palliative care early in the process would have been another valuable resource for us in the decision-making process.

Through this experience, we learned the great importance that should be placed on allowing each family to define for themselves and their child what quality of life means; what is important and valued by the family that has to make medical decisions for a child with a life-limiting condition. In my opinion, there cannot be enough emphasis on the importance of relaying the information and medical diagnosis within the context of each individual family—to empower each family to go to their unique inner strengths, knowledge, sources of spirituality, place of meaning making, and sense of knowing; to allow these decisions to arise from a place that is authentic and rooted in each family.

For the 5 weeks we lived in uncertainty without a diagnosis, we did not put our love for Will on hold. We grew deeply in love with him, just as he was, technology and all. A name did not now change that for us. They called it myotubular myopathy. We called him our son.

Parent Commentary

Will's mother has done an excellent job of identifying what parents need when receiving difficult news about their child's diagnosis or condition. Because of the level of medical intervention Will required in the NICU, his parents were aware that their son was most likely facing a life of significant challenges. Going into the meeting, they anticipated that the news would not be good. However, what they did not anticipate was the lack of preparedness, sensitivity, and empathy from this team of unknown professionals.

There are several needs mentioned by Will's mother that especially stand out to me. The first is the setting in which the information is delivered. Receiving difficult news about your child is an exceptionally emotional and stressful time for the parents. When the information is delivered in a room full of people you have never met before and will never see again, it adds to the stress. Only team members who are directly involved in the child's care (including nurses) should be present and, if possible, the physician delivering the diagnosis should be someone who is familiar with the family rather than an unknown physician. When communicating a devastating diagnosis for a child, the focus should be exclusively on the parents and should not be an invitation to fill the room with people for teaching purposes.

The other need that should go without saying is that when receiving a diagnosis, parents want current and up-to-date information on their child's disease. After parents receive a diagnosis, it is inevitable that they will search the Internet and do their own research. In this case, there was a clear disconnect given that the physician delivering Will's diagnosis was not aware that the lead researcher for the disease was located in the same institution. While this situation is likely not the norm, it is an important reminder that if the physician delivering the news of a rare diagnosis is not an expert on the disease, he or she should conduct their research before meeting with the parents, because you can be assured that the parents will do their own research after the meeting.

Will's mother also shares that palliative care should be included early in the decision-making process. I certainly agree with this, but also caution that if palliative care is introduced to the family, it is important that parents understand that palliative care does not equate to end-of-life care. I believe there is often resistance by parents to bring the palliative care team on board because they assume it means nothing more medically will be done for their child. Assuring parents that their child will continue to receive compassionate and optimal medical care while on palliative care is important.

How difficult news is delivered can have a significant impact on the parent-physician relationship and, if not handled well, can result in unintended emotional distress to the parents and a loss of trust. Preparedness (know the family and the disease), sensitivity (to the setting and the parent's reaction and nonverbal cues), and empathy are paramount when delivering a child's life-altering diagnosis to their parents.

Physician Commentary

Here is how physicians view these meetings where a difficult diagnosis is presented to families: we really want to get it right. We want to have the content experts, e.g., neurologists, present. This is truly an unusual situation where a research expert in the field was a member of the institution; he or she perhaps should have been included in this meeting. We want to include team members who have been involved with the child's care or might be in the future. In my experience, the child's primary bedside nurse(s) (those who have cared for the child the most) are included, if at all possible. But we also recognize how overwhelming the sheer number of people can be, and how intimidating. In academic medical centers, we want our trainees to be present, both to learn how to relay such information but also because they often have strong relationships with the family, or as physicians, sometimes stronger than the attending physicians at times.

Recognizing the number of attendees can be intimidating (and personally I try to limit the numbers at such meetings), it is the primary bearer of the news on whom the brunt of the burden falls—to get it right. Information needs to be delivered so families can understand. Except in rare cases, every diagnosis has a range of prognoses and options for care. That wide range should be highlighted at an initial meeting, but there should be no expectation of decisions to be made right away. Information needs to sink in, and parents have a right to consider the implications of the diagnosis and the choices for their unique circumstances and wishes. Messages of challenging diagnoses call for the maximal amount of empathy that a physician can muster. The message should always include: we will always be there for you.

A final comment about palliative care. Our society equates palliative care with hospice—it means my child is going to die. Nothing could be further from the truth. Modern pediatric palliative care teams bring a wide swath of expertise to add support to children and families in difficult situations, regardless of the prognosis. These teams can explore patients' and families' values, goals, struggles, and challenges in ways a "regular" physician simply is not trained to do. Palliative care includes physicians, advanced practice nurses, social workers, psychologists, and others who can wrap themselves around a family in a time of great need. Alas, this is a relatively young field in pediatrics, and many institutions do not yet have a robust service in place as I have described. If it does exist where you find yourself, please ask for their help.

Advocacy Is Not Anger

31

As a new palliative medicine physician in a large Children's Hospital, I quickly learned that much of my work centered on communication. I have learned many lessons from my interactions with children and their families over the years. I remember one child and his mom who taught me a valuable lesson about the challenges we face when we jump to our own conclusions about another person's emotions.

The consult call came in on a Friday afternoon. It had been a busy day and admittedly, I was ready for the weekend. The medical team was asking for help with an "angry mom." As they said those words, I started to make my own assumptions and predictions about how this encounter might go. For many reasons, anger always felt like a hard emotion to address.

The primary medical team told me about Nate, an 8-year-old, who was born with a chromosomal deletion syndrome that affected his entire body. He was unable to walk or talk and used a tracheostomy and ventilator to support his breathing. The team told me that Nate had been displaying some agitation, which they felt was going to be his new baseline. They related to me the conversations they had been having with Nate's mom. They were ready to send Nate home, but his mom was refusing. They felt she was not accepting his new baseline and had become "angry" with the medical team based on her insistence that there was something wrong with him and the medical team was just not finding it.

I headed over to see Nate and his mom. Although I did not know how the meeting would go, I braced myself for the possibility of a highly charged encounter. As I arrived to see Nate, his mom was pacing around the room and I could quickly see why the team might assume she was angry. She immediately told me "we have to do something about this," meaning Nate's agitation. I asked for more information and she described how her son had been at home—more interactive with smiles and vocalizations at times. She described her frustrations since Nate's hospitalization, feeling that his condition changed before her eyes and he now appeared uncomfortable most of the time. She spoke to me about how the team had told her this was his new baseline. She expressed her frustration as she told them repeatedly that this was

© Springer Nature Switzerland AG 2021
A. F. Schrooten, B. P. Markovitz, *Shared Struggles*,
https://doi.org/10.1007/978-3-030-68020-6_31

new, and there was something wrong. Her tone and the volume of her voice raised each time. I wondered if she was angry or if she thought talking louder or in a different tone of voice would make someone hear her concerns. I concluded our conversation by reassuring her I would speak with the team and come up with a plan to help Nate's agitation. I also told her that I could not promise we would find a reason for it.

As I left the room to go talk with the team, I could hear Nate's mom's voice telling me that we needed to do something, urging me to make her son feel better. At times in our conversation, she raised her voice to make a point. I thought about how we often assign emotions to people without really asking them what they are feeling. At that point, I decided I was falling into the same trap. I assumed she was angry, just like the team, because we had not yet been able to fix the problem or get her son back to his normal self. I realized that assuming she was angry could quickly lead to labels like "difficult mom" or "she doesn't understand his disease." Was that fair to Nate's mom or to any family member in this situation? I decided to turn around, go back into the room, and ask Nate's mom what she was really feeling.

As I walked back to the room, I will admit I questioned what I was doing. If Nate's mom really was angry, I could bear the brunt of that emotion. I had already done what I needed to do, I was not sure I had the reserve, this late on a Friday afternoon, for conflict. I remember taking a deep breath as I entered the room telling myself this was important, remembering the times I had been on the other side of this equation with my own family members.

"Hi, I was wondering if we could talk a little more about our earlier conversation," I said.

"Sure, do you have more questions about Nate's symptoms or care?" she replied. "Actually, I was hoping to talk with you more about how you are feeling."

I could see she was surprised by my inquiry and her guard was up, so I paused as I tried to figure out what to say next. I recalled one of my mentors telling me that sometimes you just have to give a name to the emotion you think you are seeing. You might be wrong, but at least it is a discussion point.

"I want to understand your perspective so I can best care for Nate and your family. It seems like you might be angry with the care team or with aspects of his care," I stated quietly, bracing myself for the answer.

"Although I'm aware that others think I'm angry at Nate's team or about his care or the situation, I'm not angry," she stated.

I was surprised by this answer. She explained to me that she was just doing the best she could to advocate for her child and be a good parent. Although she often wished the team would listen more, she felt most were doing the best they could. It was her job, she told me, to make sure that if there was a way to improve Nate's comfort or figure out why he had changed in this way, she had to see it happen. She was Nate's voice, his advocate.

As I left the room a second time, I thought about how much work families must do to advocate on behalf of their child. The old adage "the squeaky wheel gets the grease" came to mind. I felt sad that our families who advocate for what they need might be labeled as angry or difficult rather than just trying to navigate a challenging situation the best they can for their child and family. I told myself that in the future I would ask parents about their emotions rather than assigning labels. I would do better at helping them advocate for their child. I promptly found the medical team and shared this lesson learned with them as well.

Following our encounter, Nate began a new medication for his agitation and eventually returned to his more interactive and smiling self. He was able to go home and remain out of the hospital for over a year. Nate's mom continues to advocate for Nate's needs as they arise. I continue to take forward my lesson of asking and not assuming when helping my patients and families advocate for what they need.

Parent Commentary

It is interesting how we (or maybe it is just me!) will raise our voice to make sure we are heard, even though the person we are talking to is standing right in front of us. Yet, if we felt that the person is truly listening to what we are saying, my guess is that we would not feel the need to raise our voice. When you actively listen to someone, you validate what they are saying, even if you do not always agree with it. For parents who are feeling vulnerable and out of control (which is what every parent feels in a hospital setting), validation of our opinions, suggestions, and concerns regarding our child can make all the difference in how we interact with our child's care team. We know that our child's doctors only want what is best for our child and we know we really are on the same "team," however, what we know intellectually and what we feel are not always aligned if we do not feel that our voice is given the weight it merits.

It cannot be overstated that the parent knows their child best. There is so much that parents do to keep their child well and out of the hospital that is unseen and often underappreciated by the team that only sees our child when they are sick and in the hospital. We bring our child to the hospital only after we have thought of every possible explanation and used everything in our home medical arsenal to help our child feel better, and have been unsuccessful. Yes, we need your help, but we do not relinquish all of our opinions, ideas, or control when we place our child under your care.

Because there is such a short window of time that the team and the parent have together, there can be little opportunity for a meaningful discussion, especially when the parent has a different opinion from the team's consensus. Thus, the raising of one's voice. And let us be honest, as this story demonstrates, showing emotion is often the only way we can get the focused time and attention we need from our child's doctor. We are not oblivious to the labels that are attached to us when we have to push a little harder (and louder) to be heard, however, as this doctor recognizes, all those labels and emotions point to one predominant label: advocate.

When conflict arises between the medical team and the parent, whether real or perceived (i.e., anger vs. advocacy), what this story shows us is the importance of communication. Making assumptions takes no time or effort and assumptions can often be wrong. Instead, as this doctor did, make the extra effort and take the time to talk with the parent. Be a seeker of information rather than a conveyor of information and find out what the parent is thinking, how they are feeling, and why. We are much more likely to consider and accept your recommendation or conclusion if you listen to us, validate what we have to say, and then explain why you think differently. Through good communication, flexibility, and mutual respect, together we can achieve what is best for our child with minimal conflict and a better understanding of one another.

Physician Commentary

This is a very meaningful lesson for all physicians and reinforces the simple adage: first seek to understand. Do not judge. Open your mind. Put yourselves in the other's shoes. Wear their glasses for a day. Walk in their footsteps. Of course, all these watchwords should be part of our everyday communication patterns with each other, but they are especially important when voices are raised and a child's life may literally be on the line. If you do not understand the "why" behind the behavior of another, you will not be able to help them, or in this case, their child.

This is also yet another example, although it is not highlighted, that parents know their children best. Not only do they know that something is wrong, they may know precisely what is wrong, how to look for the problem, and even how to treat it. Alternatively, a physician may be less inclined to "turn over every rock" in some of these situations to look for problems since they may not even appreciate the subtle changes that parents can see. Even common pediatric conditions may not present in "textbook fashion" in many such complex children, and an open mind with an approach of curiosity is warranted. That same open mind and curiosity is how we should approach parents when they are advocating, strongly or calmly, for the most precious people in their lives.

Where Is the Doctor?

32

It is 4:30 am and I am sitting in the emergency department of our Children's Hospital desperate for some pain relief for my son, Jack. After a night of no sleep because of pain that could not be controlled by the morphine dosage prescribed by his palliative care doctor, my only option was to bring Jack to the emergency department to try and find the source of his pain and obtain some relief. With a nonverbal child suffering from a progressive neuromuscular disease, it is difficult to know where to start.

Is it the recurring kidney stones that were shown to be stable when checked just a month ago?

Is it the broken femur discovered just a few weeks ago?

His failing heart?

It was a quiet predawn morning and we were quickly ushered to a room. I handed the nurse my four-page typed document outlining Jack's history and current medical information. Fourteen years of medical history for a medically complex child includes enough events, procedures, surgeries, medications, and complications to overwhelm a seasoned doctor, let alone the resident charged with the task of obtaining Jack's medical history. I learned long ago that it is easier to write it down and update as we go along.

The resident came into the room with the document in her hand. I gave her additional details of Jack's current condition and issues with pain. I explained that he has kidney stones filling a significant portion of his right kidney despite two surgeries and an arsenal of medications prescribed to prevent stone formation. No one seemed to know why the stones regenerate other than the fact that "Jack is a very sick and complicated child." I told her that he had a CT scan a month ago and the stones appeared stable. With Jack still in his wheelchair, the resident conducted a brief exam. Based on his history of kidney stones, she ordered a CT scan along with blood work to check for infection.

Jack's weary and distant eyes conveyed the magnitude of the pain that consumed him. I needed to get him out of his wheelchair and into a more comfortable position on the bed. After the resident left the room, I pressed the call button and asked for

© Springer Nature Switzerland AG 2021   161
A. F. Schrooten, B. P. Markovitz, *Shared Struggles*,
https://doi.org/10.1007/978-3-030-68020-6_32

help to move Jack. Transferring Jack and the ventilator he is tethered to from the wheelchair to the bed is at least a two-person job. Moving him to the bed did little to relieve his pain. I pressed the call button again and asked if he could please have something for pain. There was no pillow on the bed. I asked for a pillow. Time has a way of slowing down when your child is in pain and you are at the mercy of others. After what felt like an hour, but was likely a much shorter time, the nurse returned with a pillow. As the pain continued to hold its grip on Jack, I pled, "Can he please have something for pain?" The nurse sharply responded that he was getting me the pillow I asked for and that "I can only do one thing at a time!"

I felt the sting of tears as exhaustion and frustration overwhelmed me. I wanted to say out loud, but instead silently thought to myself, "I wish you could understand that it is not my intention to be difficult or demanding. I am just desperate for my son to get some relief from his pain. My child is hurting and I need your help. I brought him here because I cannot help him. I wish I could manage all his needs at home. I tried, but this time I cannot do it alone. I do not want to be here because experience tells me that when you see my child you will only see his disability, the ventilator and the progressive disease that is slowly destroying his body. You will not see the child beneath the disease and all the equipment—the typically happy boy who can light up a room with his smile and his eyes. All he wants is to stop hurting. Can you please just help him stop hurting?"

More than an hour after being seen by the resident, the nurse placed an IV and Jack finally received something for pain. As his pain slowly eased, Jack closed his eyes and found relief in the sleep that had eluded him for most of the last 24 hours.

When it was time for the CT scan, I followed Jack to radiology. I assisted and instructed as he was transferred to the narrow table. I knew the simple misplacement of his arm or leg could result in a fracture. The radiology staff was very patient and understanding. Shortly after returning from radiology it was time for shift change. The emergency department attending physician poked her head in the room and told me that she was leaving and I should hear the results of the CT scan shortly. That was the first and only time I saw the attending physician.

As Jack slept, I was finally able to relax a bit. I kept a watchful eye on his heart rate, respirations, and oxygen saturations as the numbers streamed across the monitor on the wall. I bounced back and forth between sitting in a chair and standing at Jack's bedside in an effort to stay awake. An hour or so later, the resident came back to the room and let me know that the CT scan was consistent with the scan from a month ago and that the kidney stones were stable and did not appear to be the source of Jack's pain. She also conveyed that nothing concerning showed up in his blood work. Beyond conveying the test results, she offered nothing further before leaving the room. I wondered where we were supposed to go from here.

Did they have any ideas as to what could be causing Jack's pain?

Are there any other tests that might be helpful?

If we cannot determine the source of Jack's pain, what is the plan for pain management?

The only insight I received as to what the plan might be was when the nurse told me that if they could not find the source of Jack's pain, he would likely be admitted.

I called my husband and gave him an update. I also sent a text to our palliative care social worker to let her know what was going on. Shortly after getting my text, our social worker called. I did not get too far into the conversation before she gently asked me if I wanted to consider transitioning Jack to hospice. This was not the first time she brought up the subject of hospice to me. All the previous times my answer was adamantly "No." It had not even been a year since we transitioned Jack to palliative care after learning that his heart function had significantly declined due to progression of his disease. This time when the question was asked, I did not feel as adamant.

It had been almost a year to the day that we were in the same situation with Jack—sitting in the emergency department because of pain issues that could not be managed at home. Last year, Jack was admitted and endured a 3-week stay in the Pediatric ICU, a multitude of tests and a surgery—all of which yielded few answers and little relief for Jack. I was not convinced that another admission would give us any different results. In fact, I was not convinced of anything because I had limited information and I was not getting any guidance. We had been in the emergency department for over 5 hours and an attending had yet to come into the room to examine Jack or talk with me about what was known, what was not known, and what our options were.

I called my husband. After talking it over, we decided that we were not going to admit Jack. I called our social worker next. I told her that we were ready to transition Jack to hospice.

I have never felt so alone as I did sitting in that tiny, cramped emergency department room as Jack slept—the rhythmic clicking of the ventilator that had sustained his life the last 14 years the only thing breaking the silence. Tears fell as I looked at my weary son. Just outside our closed door was a hospital filled with medical professionals who dedicate their lives to helping children—including Jack's own palliative care doctor. Yet there was not a single doctor available to help me make the most difficult decision of my life.

Four months after that visit to the emergency department, Jack died. For the rest of my life I will question whether we made the right decision. Whether we even made an informed decision. No parent should have to make the decision to transition their child to hospice sitting alone in the emergency department without having had a single discussion with an attending physician regarding their child's history, present condition, and all available options.

Parent Commentary

Parents of medically complex children have the knowledge and acumen to handle just about everything their child throws at them. When our child is sick, we have the experience and resources to manage their care at home. We care for tracheostomies, feeding tubes, and central lines. We give round-the-clock medications and treatments. We troubleshoot and adjust ventilators. We come to the hospital only as a last resort. Our children are complex and their medical history and underlying condition can be overwhelming. But beyond the complexity, the technology, and the disease is a child who is hurting and a concerned parent who is asking for help.

The attending physician never examined Jack and never talked with his mother. It is difficult to understand why Jack was not seen by the attending physician—the physician with the most experience and the physician ultimately responsible for the care provided in the emergency department. Was it because Jack's pain was not seen as an emergency? Or because Jack could not articulate his pain? Was it because pain was to be expected given Jack's condition? A short conversation with the attending physician would have gone a long way in alleviating the uncertainty Jack's mother must live with for the rest of her life. If the attending did not feel comfortable talking about end-of-life decisions, then Jack's palliative care doctor should have been called.

Parents of medically complex children are resilient and they are knowledgeable. But they still need the support and guidance of the physicians in whose hands they place their child's care. Especially when they have to make decisions that can be the difference between their child's life and death.

Physician Commentary

This is truly an unfortunate story and on the surface, represents the failure of our pediatric health system to comprehensively manage a child like Jack. We function in our own spheres of our specialties and subspecialties and it is difficult to find one physician, or a multidisciplinary team to be "captains of the ship" with respect to caring for a child this complex. I would like to comment on two elements here, among the many that this story presents.

The first is the child's pain and the mother's cries for help. Except in rare instances, parents always know their children—particularly complex care children—better than any physician or nurse. If the mother knew Jack was in pain, he was in pain. If you could not see it in his eyes, surely the staff could see it in the mother's eyes. Short of a few conditions, there is no downside to immediately addressing the primary concern here—Jack's pain. Once his medication history has been reviewed, aggressively treating his pain should have been the number one priority. All physicians worry about the primary side effect of opioids (narcotics—which remain our most powerful pain medication), that of respiratory depression. Give enough morphine and patients can stop breathing. However, in Jack's case, he is on a ventilator already and that risk is essentially nonexistent. For too long physicians in general, and pediatricians in particular, underestimated the recognition of pain and poorly managed it. That has been changing, but the reticence to give powerful analgesic medications remains.

The second issue here is the loneliness Jack's mother felt making the decision not to admit Jack and transition him to hospice care. Palliative care medicine is emerging now in many Children's Hospitals to be a powerful force in managing complex children and their comfort needs. Palliative care is not the same as hospice—or end-of-life care—though that can be one outcome of their involvement over time. It sounds like Jack was followed by a palliative care team, but they are not often available 24/7 and there are too few physicians in this subspecialty of pediatrics. I do not know the details of their involvement with Jack, but one of the elements of care these multidisciplinary teams can and should do is planning. In Jack's case, one wonders what plans were discussed in the event he had another episode of pain that could not be managed at home. I am reluctant to speculate, but discussions about limitations of care and how to escalate comfort measures may—and I emphasize *may*—avoid the situation that this parent is describing. I say "may" because, speaking from my own experience, sometimes families are not open to discussing such contingencies. Jack's mother states that hospice had been brought up before, so it is likely that some of these discussions were held. She rightly was disappointed in the lack of the emergency department attending physician involvement, but certainly it is not the role of the ED physicians to discuss hospice with patients they do not know.

Jack had a progressive and incurable disease. That he lived and thrived for so many years is a tribute to a village of support and to his supremely dedicated parents most of all. But there was going to be an end, and it sounds like that village let Jack and his mother down by not preparing them to recognize what situations would arise that would trigger a smoother transition to purely comfort care. Having said that, I believe Jack's parents still did what they had to do; to be certain that there was not a readily "fixable" problem. It is just unfortunate that Jack's mother felt so alone in that moment in making this transition. Despite what I said about the limited role an ED attending could play here, even a physician who did not know Jack could have sat down with his mother, held her hand, and offered support and reassurance of the correctness of her decision.

Failure to Communicate

33

My smart and social 16-year-old son, Luke, was born with collagen VI-deficient congenital muscular dystrophy, which has caused progressive muscle weakness and contractures (constriction in his joints) since birth. He uses a power wheelchair to get around and his competitive nature shines through when he is playing wheelchair hockey—a game he loves and has played since he was 7 years old.

Luke is an informed and active participant in the management of his disease. He participated in one of the first clinical trials at the National Institutes of Health to gauge baseline muscle function over time in individuals affected with congenital muscular dystrophy. As part of the study, Luke had pulmonary function testing. The results were sent to our local pulmonologist who has been following Luke since he was 9 years old. Although Luke participated in the study during the summer and general information was shared after testing, the specific results of the pulmonary function test were not available to us until Luke's routine appointment with his pulmonologist several months later.

Heading into the appointment, Luke and I were both aware there had been some decline in his respiratory status. We expected he might need some adjustments to his current respiratory support, which consisted of nighttime use of a BiPAP machine that delivers breathing support through a face mask.

After completing his exam, the pulmonologist shared the results of the pulmonary function test, which confirmed our suspicions and showed a continued significant decline in Luke's lung capacity. When he asked Luke how he was feeling, Luke said he was feeling okay, but acknowledged he had been having headaches and that, in addition to using his BiPAP machine at night, he was now having to use it during the day after school.

Without any further discussion, the pulmonologist told Luke it was time he started using daytime ventilatory support in addition to BiPAP at night. When I heard this, I felt my heart skip a beat. Neither Luke nor I said anything. Breaking the silence, I asked Luke, "What do you think about that?" Without looking up from his phone, Luke adamantly said, "I'm not doing that!"

© Springer Nature Switzerland AG 2021

A. F. Schrooten, B. P. Markovitz, *Shared Struggles*,

https://doi.org/10.1007/978-3-030-68020-6_33

Acknowledging Luke's resistance to the idea, the pulmonologist assured Luke that he would not need a tracheostomy; that he could continue to use noninvasive ventilation by using a portable ventilator that would hang from the back of his wheelchair and be attached to tubing and a mouthpiece. Luke refused to make eye contact with either of us and just kept looking down at his phone.

As I listened to the exchange, or lack thereof, between Luke and his pulmonologist, I tried not to cry. While trying to process the information, I fired off questions.

"Should we get a sleep study first?"

"Would some adjustments to his overnight BiPAP settings help?"

"Is daytime ventilation the only option?"

I was not prepared to hear that Luke's health had declined to the point of needing what both Luke and I felt was an extreme intervention. Appearing somewhat annoyed that I was pushing back and questioning his recommendation, the pulmonologist responded matter-of-factly, "Luke is experiencing chronic respiratory failure and it is not going to get better."

Hearing the words "chronic respiratory failure," I felt like I had been shot. I had trouble thinking clearly. All I could think was, *Luke is going to die.* Even though I knew intellectually that what the pulmonologist suggested would help Luke, in my mind all I could imagine was his imminent death. I could not catch my breath as I looked over at Luke. He was staring intently at his phone, with his jaw set and refusing to make eye contact with me or the doctor. Luke and his pulmonologist had a good relationship, so the fact that he was not saying a word after hearing what was said was significant. He was clearly shaken by the statement.

I do not know if the pulmonologist was purposely going for the shock factor because I pushed back with questions and concerns or maybe he was short on time and needed me to grasp the severity of Luke's respiratory decline without having to engage in a lengthy discussion. But his blunt choice of words stunned me. It was all I could do to hold it together for the remainder of the appointment. We concluded the appointment by agreeing to come back for a noninvasive ventilation trial after which we would decide how we wanted to proceed.

As we approached the elevator to leave the office, I had an overwhelming sense that my conversation with the pulmonologist was not finished. I needed to speak what was on my mind while still in the moment. I was crying and upset by how such serious news was delivered. The pulmonologist had been providing care to Luke for more than 7 years. He knows me as an educated parent and zealous advocate for Luke. I felt both Luke and I deserved more patience and compassion than he displayed. I told Luke that I was going back to talk with his pulmonologist. Luke nodded and said he would stay where he was and wait for me.

I found the pulmonologist in the hallway where the nurses and doctors do their charting between appointments. He looked surprised to see me standing in front of him again, probably, in part, because I was crying. I talked to him through my tears, telling him there had to be a better way to convey the hard and unexpected news to an intelligent 16 year-old with muscular dystrophy and his mother that he needed full-time respiratory support without using the words "chronic respiratory failure." The pulmonologist looked surprised, but I kept talking. I explained that I felt my questions and concerns had been minimized and dismissed.

It was apparent from the pulmonologist's wide-eyed expression that he was caught off guard by my sudden reappearance and by what I had to say. He tried to interject a few times, but I continued to talk. I needed to get everything off my chest and convey my perspective on what had transpired during Luke's appointment and how disappointed I was. To his credit, the pulmonologist eventually stopped talking and listened. When I was finished, he seemed to recognize how poorly he handled his delivery of information about Luke's respiratory decline. Before leaving to get back to Luke, I told him I would email the nurse practitioner about scheduling the ventilation trial.

Ultimately, after trialing noninvasive ventilation, Luke agreed to use it during the day. It has made a tremendous difference in his quality of life. He no longer suffers from headaches and he has more energy.

I recently asked Luke about his recollection of the appointment. How did he feel about how his pulmonologist delivered the news of his respiratory decline? He said that at the time he did not feel there was a problem that warranted starting down the path his pulmonologist recommended, mostly because he did not yet realize his life would not improve from a respiratory standpoint. He was not prepared for the words *"chronic respiratory failure"* and felt the way his pulmonologist delivered the information was lacking in compassion. He was very scared when he heard those words. He thought "respiratory failure" meant he was dying. This was devastating to me all over again. I was heartbroken hearing that Luke thought he was not going to live much longer.

The impact of the words chosen by the pulmonologist when conveying Luke's condition may have been unintended, but the distressing feelings they invoked have not been forgotten by his patient, even many years later.

Parent Commentary

Luke and his pulmonologist appear to have a long-term ongoing doctor-patient relationship. Maybe it was because they were so familiar with each other that the pulmonologist felt comfortable conveying the news of Luke's respiratory decline in such a direct and frank manner—likely the same way he has conveyed less worrisome news to Luke and his mother over the years. Or, perhaps it was because he was running short on time that particular day and he did not have time for the questions being asked by Luke's mother. Whatever the reason, it was important to Luke, and to Luke's mother as his advocate, that Luke's pulmonologist understand that when delivering unexpected and difficult-to-hear information that affects your patient's quality of life, they needed more from him than he gave them. They needed more time, more information, and more compassion.

A physician's communication style can dramatically affect the parent/patient experience. When delivering difficult news, a little compassion goes a long way in softening the impact. It is important to give the parent and patient time to digest the information you just shared before rushing directly to the treatment options and expecting them to see things your way. Allow time and be prepared for questions and requests for clarification. Recognizing that the window of time a physician has with each patient on a busy clinic day is short, if a physician knows that he or she will be discussing a significant change in the patient's condition, if possible, try to schedule the patient's appointment at the end of the day or at a time when the physician can take extra time with the patient. It is also important to be open to the suggestions and opinions of the parent, we know our child's condition best and our input is important and invaluable.

Ask us (and our child, if appropriate) what our understanding is of the news that you just dropped on us. As intelligent and experienced as we may be, you cannot assume that we understand the nuance of the medical terminology you use to describe a condition or diagnosis. It is also important to recognize that our view of the "big picture" may be very different from your own. Luke's pulmonologist saw a noninvasive treatment option to help Luke breathe easier during the day and slow down his respiratory decline. Luke and his mother saw death staring them in the face.

In the end, Luke and his mother agreed with the pulmonologist and what he recommended was the right option for Luke. However, getting to that point came at an unnecessarily high emotional cost to Luke and his mother that could have been mitigated with a dose of compassion and a few extra minutes to listen and explain.

Physician Commentary

In the ideal world, every physician-patient/parent interaction would start with the physician asking: "What is your understanding of your condition now?" This allows the patient/parent to open the dialogue and express their understanding and concerns. The physician then can engage with the knowledge of where the patient/parent is at the time. This is particularly helpful with multiple physicians involved, as physicians may not often communicate well with each other about their mutual patients. In this case, Luke may well have been worried that his symptoms were, in fact, a sign of deteriorating respiratory function, and the physician could then have compassionately confirmed his correct concerns.

In any case, our medical jargon and terminology, which we too often throw out so casually, is either completely not understood by our patients, or we fail to recognize the weight some words have when received by nonmedical individuals. "Failure" is one such extremely loaded word. We know what we mean when we say an organ is failing—it means dysfunctional, but not necessarily dying. However, nonmedical people interpret the word failure with a great deal more weight. Perhaps the most hurtful phrase we could say to another human being (especially a teenager) is: "you are a failure." How then is being in respiratory failure different than being a failure? Luke's mother stated this outright: respiratory failure means death.

I have a colleague who is a specialist in treating children with "heart failure" and refuses to use the phrase intentionally, for these very reasons. Furthermore, definitions of organ failure are often either extremely subjective or, alternatively, determined by tiny functional alterations.

Finally, I do not lend much leeway to the suggestion of letting this doctor off the hook a bit by suggesting he was pressed for time. Who is not always pressed for time? I would argue that being compassionate and empathetic takes almost no extra time at all. "Luke, I want to confirm your concerns, that your symptoms may be a sign of needing more breathing assistance. I know this must be hard to hear. I am going to be there for you and work with you to support you to the best of my ability. Let me suggest some choices."

Four sentences may have made the difference in this encounter between the reactions Luke and his mother had and a further cementing of the therapeutic bond so vital between physicians and their patients and families.

When a Patient and Family Forever Change Your World

34

The best thing about working in the field of pediatric complex care is getting to know patients and families. What a privilege it is to establish a long-term partnership with a family and to collaborate together on how to optimize the health and wellbeing of a child with medical complexity. Of course, every patient-family relationship is so important to keep active and strong. However, there are some relationships that elevate to a higher level. I would like to tell you about one of those that developed with Will and his parents, Erin and Mark. That relationship has forever changed not only my life, but my clinical colleagues, and the health system where I practice.

Before I get into the story, I need to catch you up-to-speed on some context about me and my frame of thinking when Will's parents and I engaged. I am a general pediatrician, a hospitalist, and a health services researcher. I have focused my life on caring for children with medical complexity and investigating ways to optimize systems of care for them. That focus emerged during medical school and my residency training, when my teachers and attending clinicians encouraged me to embrace the care of complex patients and to not shy away from taking on that care. From my 15 years of clinical experience in complex care, I would like to think that I know what is best for the children and their families under my care. However, I still have a tremendous amount to learn. Each day brings a new learning experience, many of which are quite humbling.

My own children and my family members—knock on wood—have, for the most part, been healthy. They have been living their lives free of a chronic health condition or severe impairment in their functioning and wellbeing. Although I am grateful for that, I often feel like an impostor when caring for children with medical complexity and their families. To me, no clinician can truly understand what is best for these children and their families without walking in their shoes. Well, Will's parents opened up their lives to me in a way that I had never experienced before. They gave me a personalized and heartwarming, yet honest look into their

© Springer Nature Switzerland AG 2021   173
A. F. Schrooten, B. P. Markovitz, *Shared Struggles*,
https://doi.org/10.1007/978-3-030-68020-6_34

experiences and perceptions of health care with Will. They portrayed the good, the bad, and the ugly about our health-care system and then went beyond the call of duty to help fix it.

Here is how it all happened.

With federal funding from the Agency for Healthcare Research and Quality (AHRQ), I was charged to lead a multiple multidisciplinary team of anesthesiologists, surgeons, complex care pediatricians, nurses, and everyone across the care continuum from inpatient to outpatient, to optimize the health and safety of children with medical complexity as they undergo high-risk surgery, including spinal fusion for neuromuscular scoliosis. I knew from the beginning of this project that I needed big-time help from all the stakeholders involved in preparing a child for surgery and keeping them safe throughout their episode of perioperative care—that is, from the moment that surgery is considered through full recovery from the surgery, weeks to months later. Before engaging all of the clinical stakeholders, I thought it best to begin learning from patients and families who had gone through a high-risk surgery.

Enter Will and his parents. Will is now a young adult with myotubular myopathy, which is a very rare disease that impedes the ability of his skeletal muscles to contract. So, Will relies on a tracheostomy and a ventilator to breathe. Will is cared for by our Complex Care program, and his mother and father have partnered with me on past projects involving improvements in health systems for children with medical complexity. Will's mother is an internationally renowned patient and family advocate. His father is a systems engineer working in health-care industry. And I knew that Will had undergone spinal fusion surgery for neuromuscular scoliosis, which is a long, physiologically stressful surgery that often takes weeks and months for full recovery. Spinal fusion is also associated with high rates of complications. I suspected that Will's parents would have a lot to say about the project, including good ideas on how to optimize perioperative care.

I reached out to Erin and Mark to see whether they would sit down and talk with me about their perioperative experiences. I was especially interested in learning about Will's preparation for surgery, including how they orchestrated and aligned all of the specialists and other health-care team members to make sure that everyone was thinking about the potential risks of surgery and how they were alleviated. Will's parents invited me for dinner at their home. There we could sit down and talk about their perceptions and experiences and brainstorm ideas for care improvements. I carefully planned out the questions that I wanted to ask them through a semi-structured interview guide. I had four pages worth of probing questions to help spark the conversation and to elicit rich data and stories from the family. I had my tape recorder ready to record their answers and my notepad and pen ready to take notes. I was so eager to hear what they might have to say.

The day of our meeting came. They invited me into their incredible home. It was fully equipped to serve Will's needs. His room was so cool. They had all of his medical equipment (which was enough to fill a room in our intensive care unit) organized and laid out beautifully. He had a ceiling- and wall-mounted lift-and-transport system, which enabled him to move around his room and house. Despite all of this equipment, it did not dominate Will's room. Rather, Will's Red Sox and other sports paraphernalia was the centerpiece. You could easily see his personality shining through.

For an ice breaker, Will's parents offered me a local, microbrewed India Pale Ale (IPA) with a solid number of international bitter units. I gleefully accepted. They were really trying to make me feel comfortable and welcomed into their home, which I very much appreciated. We made our way to their back porch to eat and to get started thinking through things. I looked down at my notebook with all the questions that I had prepared for them. I had the questions strategically ordered. I was ready to go, nervous but excited. As my mouth opened to ask the first question, Will's mother calmly said, "Let us walk you through everything. We have a lot to say."

Without asking a single question of them, they spent the next 3 hours going deep into all of their experiences with Will's spinal fusion surgery. They started with the preoperative care, when the surgery was first considered. They explored options and approaches for surgery with several surgeons, who recommended vastly different degrees of correction for the curve in Will's spine. They performed their own risk assessment on Will. They systematically assessed every facet of his health—his co-existing chronic conditions, his indwelling medical devices, his chronic medications, etc.—including how all of these things interacted with each other. They picked up on some key risks, including how one of his indwelling medical devices required attention ahead of surgery to ensure that it was functioning properly.

Will's parents took charge of his pre-operative care, leading and directing his large health care team—that included numerous medical specialists—along the way. They put a tremendous amount of work into making sure that Will's health was the best it could be going into surgery. As true navigators, they were their son's main advocate, making sure that everything was in place for him to have a successful surgery.

They also advocated strongly and stayed very involved in Will's care while recovering in the hospital after surgery. He experienced a malfunction with his tracheostomy and ventilation equipment after surgery that required prompt attention. His parents were the first to recognize the problem since it was the same ventilator and humidification system used at home. They continued to speak up about it until it was remedied. They felt comfortable in situations of discordance in perceptions of Will's health between themselves and Will's health-care providers. If they were worried about something that the providers were not, then they persistently—yet politely—nudged and prompted the health-care team until appropriate action occurred.

I remember thinking, "My goodness. There is so much to learn from these experiences and so many things to fix with perioperative care for children with medical complexity." But before I could express that to the family, they calmly mentioned, "And we have a set of solutions to test that we think will be very helpful. Let's talk about how to implement them together."

I was blown away. I looked down at the tape recorder to make sure that it was working properly. The batteries had run out of power at some point along the way. There was no time to change them. Will's parents continued on!

I texted my wife at that point with the, "Honey—I'll be home later than expected. Don't wait up for me. Kiss the boys for me. Love you (emoji),"—line.

Will's parents understood fully that different families may have different levels of comfort and skills when helping to prepare their children for a major surgery. Certainly, some families may not feel empowered to do that. They understood that to create a highly reliable system of care for children with medical complexity undergoing high risk surgery, a safety net in place was needed to ensure that every child received a comprehensive evaluation of their health and that someone was designated who could step up and take charge of the perioperative care management. Their perceptions resonated with me because when a surgical need arises for a child with medical complexity, problems with their existing care management are often exposed, and these problems can elevate the child's risk for experiencing perioperative adverse events.

Care management is the oversight and support of all the health care delivered across the care continuum by all of the child's health-care providers to ensure that (1) valid health assessments occur for the children, (2) best treatment plans are derived, and (3) the plans are implemented in a high-quality way. High-quality care management—we hope—leads to the optimization of the child's health. Unfortunately, lots of children with medical complexity undergoing high-risk elective surgeries do not have strong care management. They do not have someone who is taking charge of their child's health care and working with all the providers, including specialists, primary care, therapists, home care providers, etc., to stay on top of their care and their health problems.

Just think about the health-care team of a child with medical complexity who has 20 different providers involved in the child's care. Each provider is focused on their particular specific area of expertise. Neurology is thinking about epilepsy. Cardiology is thinking about a dilated aortic root problem. Hematology is worried about coagulation. Pulmonary is worried about lung function. And all the providers are doing a great job thinking about those things, but there is not a point person or a clinician who is looking across all these problems to make sure that comprehensively the child is getting what they need and that nothing is being overlooked. Unfortunately we know from the national survey of children's health that up to 40% of children with medical complexity do not have a clinician taking charge to manage their care. The reasons for this are disheartening. It takes too much time and effort to manage their care, and this care management is not reimbursed well. Many primary care clinicians feel overwhelmed and do not feel like they have the clinical proficiency to manage care for children with medical complexity. And there may not be local access to a complex care program that could be a wraparound service to offer care management for these children.

Will's parents described the preoperative impact of not having Will's care managed well going into surgery. There is a last-minute scrambling of preoperative clearances that have to occur to get the children ready for surgery. That leads to increased stress for families and clinicians. This can all lead to surgery cancellation and delays. Especially during COVID-19 times, now we have seen how challenging it can be to find operating room time and bed availability in our intensive care unit settings when surgeries have to be rescheduled. Unmanaged care also has an impact on postoperative care. If there is no one on the outpatient side who can provide a good sign out to the inpatient providers, then they receive a deficient handoff during transitions with very little instructions for contingency planning and anticipatory guidance. This places hospital providers at risk for inducing harm with ordering of chronic medications, overlooking critical medical equipment and supplies that are used in the outpatient setting (especially from the respiratory standpoint), and not understanding the child's baseline health enough to detect early warning signs of demise.

I was in awe of the depth and scope of information Will's parents shared with me over the course of those 3 hours. I also realized that I had not touched my dinner. I thanked Will's parents for their help and we made plans to continue collaborating.

They became front-and-center as full partners in our project team that was ready to re-engineer perioperative care for high-risk surgeries in children with medical complexity so that the children and their families experience the safest, most reliable, patient-and-family-centered, and successful transit through the pre-, intra-, and postoperative phases of care. We integrated health system engineers, health services researchers, and clinical stakeholders (surgeons, anesthesiologists, general pediatricians, specialists, nurses, administrators, etc.) to design and implement the ideal perioperative workflows that would best serve the patients and families.

Will's parents were the prime catalysts for the design and vision of the project. They have been full partners throughout, spending 5+ hours weekly generating ideas and implementing feasible solutions to improve care. They helped solicit real-time feedback from 50+ other patients and families through interviews at surgery and after hospital discharge. That work uncovered new issues with care that led to the care re-design. In addition, they partnered closely with parent Blyth Lord and her national Courageous Parents Network (CPN), an online education hub to assist families of children with medical complexity with challenging medical decisions, including whether to pursue spinal fusion. They also invited our team's nurse practitioner to present this qualitative research at a national conference hosted by MTM-CTM Family Connection—the non-profit Mark and Erin founded for Will's rare disease.

Because of Will's parents willingness to meet with me, share the details of their experiences and offer up real solutions, together we engineered seven core processes into perioperative care for children with medical complexity: (1) proactive communication from the surgeons to the child's other providers about the need for spinal fusion; (2) patient chart review and phone call by a complex care general pediatrician and advanced practice nurse (APN) (who is also the parent of two children who underwent spinal fusion) for screening of past medical history, quality of life, and functioning; (3) outpatient visit for comprehensive health assessment with identification of risks, shared decision-making about surgery, and perioperative planning; (4) multidisciplinary team meeting to assess whether to proceed with surgery and finalize surgical readiness; (5) standardization of intra-operative antibiotics and irrigation procedures; (6) postoperative, inpatient consultative visits by the complex care pediatrician and APN to assist with postoperative health issues and hospital discharge planning; and (7) post-discharge follow-up with the family to monitor recovery and elicit suggestions for further improvements. Evaluation of these efforts has shown better preparation for surgery, decreased complications, faster recovery, and improved patient-and-family satisfaction with care.

I am and will forever be grateful to Will's parents who catalyzed these improvements. They changed not only my world, but the world of children with medical complexity, their families, and their clinicians when a perioperative need arises. We need more patient-and-family engagement like this throughout the health system for children with medical complexity to ideally position all of the on-going improvement initiatives for optimal effectiveness. Partnering closely with patients and families throughout that process—not just through a single, isolated meeting—is the way to go. I am so grateful that Will and his parents have been patient with me, taking the extra time to teach and mentor me along the way. I cannot thank them enough for their help.

Parent Commentary

This story is *the* model for parent-physician collaboration in the care of medically complex children: asking us for our input, listening to us, valuing what we have to say, and partnering with us to create a plan of care for our child. The collaboration in this story resulted in significant improvements that will benefit many children, not just this family's son. While not every doctor-patient/parent relationship will provide an opportunity for the level of change these parents and physician brought about, every relationship is an opportunity for collaboration, and that is all we really want—a partnership with our child's doctors.

One of the prevailing themes throughout this book is that parents want to know that someone is on their side. What that means is, we need and appreciate the doctor who has an understanding (or takes the time to gain an understanding) of what is involved in caring for a medically complex child and who is willing to advocate for us and help us navigate the challenges and roadblocks we face in the care of our child. Ideally, every child would have access to a complex care team—a multidisciplinary team that serves as the point of contact for the coordination of care for our child. It was both surprising and disappointing to hear from this physician that as many as 40% of children with medical complexity do not have a doctor in charge of managing their care.

When my son was discharged from the hospital with a trach, ventilator, G-tube, and an undiagnosed neuromuscular disorder, he was cared for by no less than six subspecialists. At that time, there was no such thing as a complex care team available to assist with the coordination of his care, so the burden fell almost entirely on me. But that was over 20 years ago. Fortunately, because of the growing number of medically complex children, more Children's Hospitals are establishing complex care teams. However, based on the data provided in this story, there is still a lot of work to be done to make sure every child and every family has the support they need.

This story gives me hope. It is also an invitation for parents to find that doctor (or health-care team) you can partner with, and for doctors to find that family they can partner with. We need each other and we are out there—parents *and* doctors recognizing a need and wanting to make a difference in the care of this unique and growing population of children. Working together, we can make meaningful improvements in the delivery of health care to our children, as this story so profoundly illustrates.

Physician Commentary

This is an extraordinary story of parent-physician collaboration that has led to systems changes for future patients, not just the child in this story. If only every medically complex child could have one coordinating physician to direct the virtual orchestra needed to care for such children, that would be a huge achievement. We have an amazing Complex Care team at our hospital and frankly, I do not see how our most complicated patients could receive the coordinated care they do without this team. The burden of coordinating care among a dozen specialists should not fall upon a parent alone.

We have discussed in this book the critical bond of trust that physicians and parents must make to enable parents to be active partners in their child's care. In most cases, building that bond does not take the skills of a world-class communicator, but it does take time. Time is the most limited resource in the lives of most physicians, as administrative burdens (including documentation hurdles in our electronic health records), regulatory oversight, and an unending drive for more efficiency, has exposed the business of medicine for what it sadly is, a business. I do not believe many families of such children recognize the tremendous burdens these changes have placed on physicians. We physicians did not recognize the weight of these changes for a long time, as they have built up gradually over years. We are like the proverbial frog in the kettle, who if dropped into boiling water would leap out immediately, but because the temperature is increased slowly over time, is unable to escape before it is too late.

I do not mean to catastrophize the situation or make excuses for physicians. I am just trying to break down the dichotomy that a doctor is either empathetic and listens well or they do not. It is a spectrum and the forces moving behind the scenes to minimize physician-patient/parent time are powerful. The lesson from this story, to me, is that despite the hurdles, one physician and one family can make a difference together. Although here we learn of a true systems change being implemented, every time a physician learns from a child and their parents, future patients can benefit from the impact on the physician.

Respect: A Two-Way Street

35

My husband and I knew our son would have a serious disability when he was born. In the sixteenth week of my pregnancy, we received the diagnosis of spina bifida. His was specifically called a myeloschisis—the severest form. His brain abnormalities were clear on ultrasound. He was unresponsive on all tests and we knew there could be a difficult outcome ahead. Yet we hoped, we prayed, and we believed in our hearts that maybe the prognosis would be better than expected.

As it turned out, when Miles was born things were worse than we had imagined. He spent his first 5 months in the ICU hooked up to machines. He had eight brain surgeries, including a high-risk Chiari 2 decompression surgery when he was 12 weeks old. I lived in the hospital, away from my 2-year-old son who was still nursing at the time. I pumped milk for my sons around the clock, was delusionally tired, and rarely ate. However, what stands out the most from that time was the coding. I watched Miles code and be brought back to life countless times during those first months of his life. He had to be bagged with oxygen hundreds, if not thousands, of times. I remember one time he coded at night and it was chaos. The doctor ran in frantically and suddenly a dozen people were around him, working on him for what felt like forever. My husband and I dropped to our knees and looked at each other because it was all beyond words. And yet, our Miles was brought back to life over and over and over again.

We adjusted to a very new normal when we brought Miles home to live with us. It was thrilling to cuddle him, feed him, and not have to ask permission to be his caregivers. Because Miles had a trach and was ventilator dependent, we depended on nurses to be in our home around the clock. We no longer had a private life. Those first few months he was home were so special and I remember feeling utterly grateful and completely terrified at the same time. The chaos did not slow down because Miles continued to code constantly. His brain abnormality would cause his brainstem to essentially "turn off." The sound of alarms blaring throughout the day was typical as I would run over and stabilize him. Sometimes I would be in the middle of cooking dinner, sprint to him, begin performing CPR, bring him to life, get him through a grand mal seizure from lack of oxygen, and then continue cooking dinner.

© Springer Nature Switzerland AG 2021

A. F. Schrooten, B. P. Markovitz, *Shared Struggles*,

https://doi.org/10.1007/978-3-030-68020-6_35

This pattern seemed stable to us, but his specialists were not as comfortable with our day-to-day routine. A few days before his first birthday, we took Miles to see the pulmonologist. While they were weighing him, he coded. His home nurse and I calmly began CPR. The clinic team that ran in to see what was occurring were not as calm. The words, "I can't believe you guys do this every day," were echoed again and again. We were admitted straight to the PICU even though his status was completely baseline. I felt they were overreacting. In hindsight, I realize I was under-reacting because I was living in a state of constant crisis.

The hospital stay following the event at the pulmonologist's office was about a week. Miles had at least 13 codes during that admission. Yet between each episode, he was a smiling, bubbly, happy baby. When he was doing well, the floor doctor would move us out of the PICU because "this kid looks completely fine." Then Miles would code and we would be sent right back. The lack of consistency and communication, coupled with lack of sleep, was frustrating and exhausting for me. After an extensive brain MRI, I got a visit from the neurosurgical resident. He was about my age and had an extremely arrogant demeanor. His bedside manner did not fit the circumstance well. While I am usually quite laid back, I immediately felt tension rise between myself and the resident.

He began with, "Your son needs something called a Chiari 2 decompression," and then went on to explain the surgery in overly simplified detail, not knowing or asking what my level of understanding was in regard to Miles' condition or the surgery he needed. He finished with, "We can do the surgery tomorrow morning."

I told him, "As I'm sure you know, Miles has already had that surgery and it did not benefit him. It was also very painful and a difficult recovery so I am not sure yet that I want to move forward. I need to talk to my husband and think about this."

He did not like that I was not immediately aligning with his plan of care and proceeded to explain the surgery to me while raising his voice, "Your son's brain is like a car crushed up against a wall. You should want that car to move away from that wall. If this were my child, I would be getting the surgery. I would not even question it. You don't seem to understand the severity of this and I am trying to explain it to you."

"I do understand. Trust me. If you only knew what this last year has been like. Also, this is my child, and he has been through a lot." I asked him, "Can you guarantee me that my son will wake up from surgery tomorrow morning?"

Of course, he could not guarantee anything (no one can), but told me it was his job to explain why the surgery was necessary and should be done. For a moment I felt like I was about to give the winning argument in a courtroom after battling the expert witness who should know much more than me. I explained that as a parent I am part of the decision-making team and it is the doctor's job to give me all the medical data and make a recommendation, not to persuade me to do what sounds good to him. Our conversation concluded with me telling him that I wanted some time to think about the decision. As I would learn in years to come, there would be many instances where I would not agree with the plan of care because my child is incredibly complex and the plan is never straightforward.

The doctor left the room at the same time my mentor from church entered with Chick-Fil-A in hand. Before I had a chance to eat, the Chief of Neurosurgery walked into the room. I knew him well and he had a much gentler approach when discussing options. He told me the decompression surgery was an option, but not a very good one because studies show that second decompressions are not extremely successful. There was no great explanation as to why Miles was coding all of the time. Maybe he would outgrow it over time, maybe not. This doctor agreed with my choice to think about it as long as I needed to. Though he added, "If you go home to think, we should send Miles home on comfort care. One of these days you may not be able to bring him back. We can have a team help you through that."

Hearing those words, my heart shattered into a million pieces and a piece of my happiness left my body. My son was going to be placed on hospice the day after his first birthday. In one way, I was not surprised, and in another my body went into total shock. I could not say much. I could not cry. I just stared at my perfect little angel baby in the hospital bed while I choked down cold chicken strips. I felt totally numb and just needed to process everything.

My mentor and I prayed. I called my husband. I rocked my child. I wondered how this was my life. We met the hospice team the next day, but it was all a blur. I remember wondering when anyone would offer me a hug, a tissue, or look me in the eyes. I felt that I was building a reputation as a "difficult" mom instead of being seen as a completely brokenhearted human. It all seemed so unfair.

My son was on hospice for an entire year as I continued to bring him back to life constantly. Because he kept living, he graduated to palliative care when he was 2 years old. He is now 5 years old and starting kindergarten. His baseline status is still extreme, but Miles is with us, he is loved, he is happy, and that is fundamentally all a parent can ask for.

So much of my learning experience with Miles prepared me for my third son, who was also born with spina bifida. He is 3 years old and has had nine brain surgeries already. When I look back on the week Miles was placed on hospice, I wish that I only remembered the compassionate Chief of Neurosurgery that gently laid out the options, gave me credit for my knowledge, and included me in the plans. Yet as humans often do, I remember the resident that made me feel belittled and angry. He seemed to see my son as an interesting case instead of a human being. He was not seeing the entire picture, that there was a life behind the surgery he was proposing. A life that could be lost or suffer more damage. And parents who were suffering greatly. To be honest, in the hundreds of times I have been in the hospital with my sons since then, I feel my muscles tense when a resident walks into the room. I have met the same version of that resident neurosurgeon many times again, just with a different face and nametag. In my experience, residents seem to be overworked and under-compassionate.

Respectful communication is really valued by parents of medically complex kids. Invite me into the dialogue and ask my opinion, or at the very least, respect my concerns. In our world, we have been forced to become experts in a field we did not choose. I dare to say that I have performed advanced CPR on a coding patient more times than most doctors. I do not need a trophy for that, but it would be nice to hear every once in a while, "Good job mom. You are clearly doing your best and have gone to great lengths for your child." I can see how a neurosurgical resident wants to feel some respect for their years of grueling work to get where they are. But so do I.

I often ask when we get admitted, "which doctor will be my son's champion of care?" They never know what I am talking about. What I mean is, when everything hits the fan, who do I go to? Who is on our side? Who helps me communicate? Ideally, I would love for this person to be a "medical parent" employed by the hospital to be *my* advocate. If you ask me, this is the missing piece of the communication puzzle, and, in an ideal world, this person would be available to every parent when their exceptionally complex kid is admitted to the hospital.

Parent Commentary

There are several important messages in this story that stand out to me. The first is that of a parent needing to have their point of view and opinions about their child's condition or the proposed plan of care considered and respected. Yes, it takes up a physician's valuable time and energy to listen to us, however, we have earned the right to the benefit of a physician's time and energy. I know some will say that we do not need to "earn" a physician's time and energy, that it is something every patient and parent should receive. Nevertheless, I think it is important to share our perspective.

We know physicians have years of formal education under their belt, have endured long hours during their residency and fellowship training, have encountered challenging and difficult patients and families, and have had many patient experiences that we know nothing about. We understand that you have worked long and hard to acquire the knowledge that you bring to us when talking to us about our child's condition or treatment plan. We respect that, or at least we should.

What we bring to you when talking to you about our child is the knowledge that comes from more sleepless nights than we can count watching every rise and fall of our child's chest, managing a ventilator, clearing our child's airway for hours on end, bagging our child back to life, administering around the clock medications; we have exhaustively researched our child's disease or condition, found the experts, sent emails, made phone calls; we have experienced a level of heartache, trauma, hope, and love that only a parent can feel for their own child.

As this parent shares, we never wanted admission to this world of rare diseases, medical terminology, technology, procedures, and surgeries—but here we are. When you find yourself in a discussion with a parent who is impatient, frustrated, angry, or disagreeable, please pause and consider (or imagine) all we have been through with our child up to that point. If we do not agree with you, it is not personal, it is because we know that, ultimately, we are the ones who have to live with the consequences and emotional toll of every decision made for our child. Trust us—we have the most at stake.

I also love the suggestion of having a parent advocate when we are inpatient with our child. We say repeatedly that we are our child's best advocate—and we are. However, we are also an exhausted advocate and there is nothing more energy sapping than being in a hospital with your child. I could not agree more with this parent about how helpful it would be to have someone available to advocate for us. How helpful it would be to have someone whose only job is to ask us what we need for our child and push to make it happen. This would be especially valuable when it comes to pain management—probably one of the most challenging and confrontational experiences of hospital life with our child. While it is unlikely we will see a "parent advocate" position added to the hospital care team anytime soon, it is worth highlighting this need. And yes, ideally, that person would be a parent who has "lived the life" and has a true understanding of what parents need. Although, I personally cannot imagine having the energy to get back in the ring to "take on" the challenges parents encounter when they are in the hospital with their child.

Physician Commentary

It is said that the most compassionate members of the medical profession are medical students. Eager and bright-eyed, they come into the field full of empathy and a zeal to help people. Sadly, it seems, after years of grueling training (though the rules are lightening the slog), many young physicians have had their hearts hardened, at least a bit. Young physicians are also the least confident, and as a defense mechanism, can present themselves as the precise opposite: overconfident. When it comes to listening to the wisdom of parents of medically complex children, I feel that my generation of physicians has not done enough to transfer this simple line of advice: trust the parents as the experts with their children.

However, parents must also recognize that in nearly every situation where a resident or fellow presents a plan to the family (particularly surgical plans), he or she has not come up with the idea on their own. Trainees are often tasked to obtain parental consent for procedures that have been deemed proper by the attending physicians. Again, this too is another area where my generation may have let our trainees down; by not modeling this behavior well enough. Consent is a process, not an event. It should not be a task to check off a list, and certainly not when it comes to children with complex needs. Trust must be established so the family knows the physician understands the child and the parents understand the physician. What is the shared mental model of the problem? What are the options? What are the risks and benefits of the options? What is the parent's understanding of the situation and choices, and how does their experience with their child help inform the physician and therefore the mutual decisions to be made?

With respect to a parent advocate, this is a fascinating idea. There are versions of this model in some institutions. An ombudsperson can function as a mediator when there is disagreement. Hospitals have "Patient Relations" teams whose sole purpose is to listen to families and advocate for them. This parent though is asking "which doctor will be my son's champion of care?" In our complex world of subspecialists, there is often no "captain of the ship" that can coordinate care in a meaningful fashion. In the ICU, the pediatric intensivist should ideally play this role. Our hospital and others have developed "Complex Care" teams that function similarly and have the advantage of coordinating care across the care continuum; from the ICU to hospital ward to home. In Pediatrics, I feel, we have heard the plight of these families and are at least taking some steps to remedy what can be rather chaotic. But we can and should do better.

Part IV

Hope

Sometimes hope is a radical act, sometimes a quietly merciful response, sometimes a second wind, or just an increased awareness of goodness and beauty. –Anne Lamott

Persistence of Hope: A Story in Two Acts

36

Act 1

You can never predict the things you remember from the days that change your life. It was a warm Georgia day and, despite it being December, we had not yet put up decorations for the holiday. I remember the way the sun came in through the windows, that glimmer that sparks when the light through a window reflects off the dust in the air. I remember the look on my mom's face, well into labor as she left the house for the hospital, the look of knowing something was wrong but hoping against hope that everything was fine; the feeling when your heart sinks knowing things are about to change forever. I remember feeling scared but not knowing why, not knowing that was the last day of my innocence.

I was 16 and thought myself an adult. I was the oldest of six children and we were expecting the seventh. I loved being a part of a big family and we were all excited to welcome my sister Anna into the fold. During my mother's pregnancy, Anna had so much personality. In retrospect, that was foreboding. Looking back now I wonder if it was her way of making her mark on the world, perhaps somehow knowing her life would be too short.

I do not remember being told she had died. That surprises me to this day. Did someone tell me? Did I pick up on some nonverbal clue that something bad had happened? Did I somehow intuitively know, putting together the heaviness in the air as my parents left for the hospital? To this day I still cannot remember, but I remember the fallout. I remember screaming at God, angry at how cold He felt that day. I remember seeing my dad broken and speechless. I remember holding my sister, so beautiful yet so heart breaking. Never having taken a breath in this world it was as if something pure had been preserved in her. I remember knowing the world would never be the same.

This story is not about my grief or how we overcame, although that is a big part of my journey. This story is about how after Anna's death hope persevered in the darkest moments. I would have never acknowledged hope in the years following her

© Springer Nature Switzerland AG 2021   189
A. F. Schrooten, B. P. Markovitz, *Shared Struggles*,
https://doi.org/10.1007/978-3-030-68020-6_36

death, but it was there. No one in my family could have named it, but deep inside we had the hope to honor my sister's legacy.

Two years after her death, our pain remained, blunted but there. Hope entered the scene in the form of a phone call. My parents, who were exploring becoming a medically fragile foster home, received a call that would once again change our lives. A baby named Jordan had been born, described as abandoned, alone in the hospital. His medical needs were such that few were willing to care for him, and at the age of 10 months old he had been in the hospital all his life. We all knew that we could not leave him abandoned. What became a large part of my family narrative was solidified that day: Jordan was a baby who needed a family and we were a family that needed a baby. The unspoken gift my sister gave us was the desire to take a leap of faith, to look past our insecurity, and embrace my brother. Later he would be joined by Sam, another child with medical needs. Together they helped form my sister's legacy.

One of the first lessons you learn when you join the medically fragile community is the world at large struggles to understand that lives lived differently do not translate to "less than." Well-meaning people testified to us "how we were so special" for "taking on" my brothers. I could not disagree more with this statement. My brothers are the greatest gift in my life and in the same way I care for my toddler without medical needs now, we cared for Jordan and Sam's needs. What people do not realize is that those well-meaning statements only serve to isolate families and kids navigating medical complexity. They miss the beauty and the vibrancy that our lives contain, that my brothers' lives contain. While they were giving sympathetic glances, they missed my brothers dancing, laughing, and having a perspective on the world few people possess.

Most of all though, they missed an even greater truth, a realized hope, a healing of fractured families, our healing of the loss of a child and my brothers' healing of loss of a parent. We healed each other. My brothers brought a joy to me and my family that we long thought was gone. That smoldering hope, once hidden, was now dancing in the hallways with sounds of my brothers intentionally removing their monitors (so we could come restart Sesame Street), one of them laughing through his trach, and steps forward in both of their medical care that we never believed would be possible.

I was in college by this point and commuted so I could be the second caregiver for my brothers. Those within our medically fragile tribe understand how important that second caregiver can be. We had highs and lows. I cut my teeth on learning how to replace tracheotomy tubes, G-tubes, and giving medications to two awesome toddlers who would figure out ways to mischievously interfere with their medical technology. I was also there when we almost lost Sam from pneumonia. I remember being in the ER as he suddenly changed, breathless, tired, one moment awake, the next moment not responding. I remember being there as they whisked him to the trauma bay, placing masks on him to prevent an inevitable intubation that would lead to weeks in the PICU.

Fortunately, this story ended with Sam recovering and thriving. I know all too well from Anna's death that recovery was not always the rule. Hope prevailed in my brothers' stories and to this day they are thriving and growing into amazing young men. During those first few years though for me, hope took another form. As I learned how to care for them and witnessed the difference their nurses, doctors, and providers made in my brothers' daily lives, I had the hope that one day I too could impact the lives of kids, much as they had impacted my brothers.

Act 2

You can never predict the things you remember from caring for a patient: the kind but firm advocacy of a patient's mom, holding someone's hand as they say goodbye to those they love, the stories of overcoming a poor prognosis, strength beyond human capabilities, seeing a kid not able to talk convey more joy to you than words could ever express. That is the world I find myself walking today.

The hope that Anna, Jordan, and Sam gave me grew into something I never foresaw. Despite my desire to avoid a long education (never say never), I found myself in medical school, then residency, and then fellowship. I learned the importance of sitting down during rounds, asking open-ended questions, and finding a way to connect on a human level with my patients. My path led me into pediatric palliative care, a place looking back in retrospect could have been my only destination.

I find myself sitting in a room with a mother and her son Timothy. Timothy shows the scars of battle, one that he had fought and was fighting valiantly. He had been born with severe congenital hydrocephalus, and as a result was unable to communicate most of his needs and had limited control of his body. His limbs with muscles tightened, he is barely able to move but still has a strength beyond imagination, and a spirit stronger than most realize. His face appears tired, but in spite of this his life still shines through. He is in the hospital with pneumonia, the fourth admission in the last 6 months. As I sit there visiting with him and his mother, she invites me into their journey, how he has defied odds and overcome so much, how they have built their life to make each day its best. She shares how his sister singing to him makes his eyes light up, how when he is in the hospital his spirit seems sad, and how she worries at night that this is all too much for him. I recall the worries shared with me by his medical team, concerns about quality of life, worries about decline, all important things to reflect on and I can tell these are also important to Timothy's mother. I balance these worries though with my own experience, recognizing that those outside of this experience can easily presume lack of joy when there is an abundance. I find myself open to follow the family's lead. She shares that she has been told "he is at a new baseline" that "he may never be the same again." She knows his body has been through so much. Over time his body has battled infection after infection, each time recovering, but each time becoming a bit frailer, more open to the next infection. This time he is sicker than the last. She notices that he has been in the hospital more the past 6 months than he has been home, and this admission he spent time in the PICU, somewhere he has not been in several years. I confess I notice this as well, and share some of her worries, but I also know the spirit of children and hope that we find ourselves where we once were. She says to me "I just want to see him light up once more while his sister sings." We determine to follow his lead and listen to what he is telling us.

The heaviness in the air lingers for a minute, then she says "do you want to see some videos of him before this admission?" Together we watch as he lights up the screen with smiles and laughter. Timothy was never able to speak but he did not need words. He found a melody of his own, and I might offer it was more beautiful than the finest symphony. I am reminded of my own world growing up. The laughs through tears, the times people pitied us and missed the joy. It is like visiting the Grand Canyon and remarking how sad it is that there is so much rock.

I am reminded that, despite pain, there is hope and joy. Fortunately, Timothy recovers and makes it back home laughing and smiling, and hope is once more present. Months later, I visit Timothy at home for a medical home visit. There is nothing more sacred to me than being invited into someone's home and witnessing the ways life has been celebrated. I find myself experiencing nostalgia looking at the medical stations in the home, recognizing the systems developed on the kitchen counters that for others seem off, but for us, for those who have lived this life, they are as functional as having a coffee station. I sit there with his mother as we remark at how happy we are to see him home. As we sit talking, we both notice his sister, stroking his face and singing as he lights up the room. The moment is not lost on us as we share a quiet smile. Hope can take our darkest days and bring out joy when we least expect it.

I do not remember the first time I felt joy after my sister's death. I do not remember the first time I felt safety from my brothers' illnesses. But I do remember those doctors who were our champions of hope. They asked for pictures and videos of the good days and helped us believe we could get back to that place. They recognized the importance of small victories and that something as simple as a spark in your loved one's eyes can be momentous. They sat in the silence with us when we just needed to know we were not alone.

Often in medicine, we mistake our role as being limited to educating and informing. However, champions follow the family's lead, letting them guide the conversation and set the pace. They unite with the family's hopes, while also giving the space to express the juxtaposition of joy and lament. Most of all, these champions see the gift and value of hope. When others see darkness and aim to prognosticate, they ask "How can we help you fulfill your hope?" And on dark days, they follow the family's lead, never forcing them to see the light of hope but gently reminding them of its presence.

My sister and brothers were my awakening to hope. Timothy and those like him have strengthened its influence and importance in my practice. He and his mother remind me that sometimes my strongest prescription is seeking out their hope rather than prescribing a medication. I realize now that I too am a hope bearer. I too have the crucial responsibility to sit quietly alongside those I serve, learn their story, and search for that quiet glimmer of hope. I cannot help but smile at the beautiful symmetry of this truth, having once been the one seeking hope, and now being among those cultivating hope. Whether we are there to restore more life or help say goodbye, we should aspire to champion this spirit, moving from hope being hidden in the corner of the room, to one day running and singing down the halls. This is the least I can do to honor the legacy of my sister and impact of my brothers.

I wish this dance was intuitive, but what I have learned from my sister, my brothers, Timothy, and all my patients is that it takes intention. I recall once sitting with a resident. She asked me "why?" Why did I choose to practice a side of medicine that at times can be so heartbreaking? My answer I think surprised her. "Hope." I shared with her Timothy's story and even my own. We should all remember that what we see at first blush is not often the truth, that hope never fails, and if you are open to it, many times you find it in the most surprising places. I shared with her the important art of asking, "What are you hoping for?" "Tell me about your child." "What makes them light up?" These are questions doctors ask far too infrequently but are so crucial to empowering hope. This is the least I can do to honor the stories and legacies of all the children like Timothy that I get the privilege to meet.

Hope is always present, you just have to be open to it. It is my core belief that this is the heart of medicine. You never know what you are going to remember. The things I do remember such as Timothy's smile, my brothers' laughter, and the countless others who I have witnessed find hope, remind me that hope has the power to create joy in the most unexpected places. And my privilege is to help give voice to that hope.

Parent Commentary

One of the most common sentiments felt by parents of children with chronic, complex needs is that doctors simply have no clue. They do not understand us or have any understanding of all that is involved in caring for our child. When it comes to living life with our child, doctors generally do not have any understanding of what challenges us, what we hope for, what brings us joy, what we need, what we do not need. More than anything, we want to be understood, yet we know that it is impossible for anyone—not just doctors, but also our own family and friends, to understand what our life is like if they have not walked in our shoes. The doctor in this story has the rare perspective of having shared experiences with his patients' families. He has personally experienced the same challenges and joys. He has a true understanding of our home life and our hospital life.

This doctor is a unique voice of hope—both as a family member and as a doctor. He knows the power of hope and the importance of being a champion of hope for his patients and their families. He is also the exception, not the rule, when it comes to the doctors we encounter in the care of our child. Through sharing his story and applying what he learned from his own family and experiences, this doctor can speak to and, more importantly, be heard by his colleagues in a way that parents cannot. This doctor took the gifts of perspective and hope that his sister and brothers gave him and he is paying it forward as both a teacher of hope and a bearer of hope. As a parent, I am grateful for his message of hope—grateful that he speaks it and he lives it.

Physician Commentary

You do not meet physicians every day that (a) have walked in the shoes of the parents of medically complex children, and (b) write this eloquently. I love the questions this physician asks: "What are you hoping for?" "What makes them light up?" As pediatricians, we try hard to return our ill patients to their "baseline," but often we fail to really find out what that means. Especially for nonverbal children, just understanding better about how they communicate, and what is the relationship like between the child and the family members. I think at every one of these encounters, parents should show a 2-minute video of their child while at home, happy and bringing happiness to others.

I think physicians struggle with the desire to provide hope while being realistic at the same time. We are obligated to provide a truthful assessment of a condition, explaining the range of possible outcomes that could be expected. Perhaps therein lies the key. Our ability to prognosticate is like predicting the future. It is imperfect at best. Hope can live and breathe in this space of uncertainty about outcomes, particularly if the physician and the parent collaboratively partner to strive for that very best possible outcome. I cannot count the number of times that a patient was not expected to survive a condition, only to find them beating the odds, sometimes with surprisingly positive outcomes. Even if, in our heart of hearts, we find it difficult to consciously offer hope, at the very least, we can endeavor to not take it away from a family.

Can I Offer You Advice?

37

Gia Grace is our third and final baby, completing our family. Immediately following her birth, we knew something was not right; her little feet were flopping, her hands were balled into tiny fists, her oxygen levels were low and, most notably, she had no cry. She was transferred from the delivery room to the NICU where she spent her first week of life. We were no strangers to the NICU; our first daughter spent several days in the exact same NICU for issues with oxygen, so our level of concern was relatively low at first. However, within a few days it became clear Gia's issues were not temporary. Fear overcame us when the medical staff began discussing the need to transfer Gia to the local Children's Hospital due to the complexity of her symptoms and level of specialized care she required. Being a Registered Nurse, I knew at that moment her condition was serious and I found myself crying while the NICU nurses held my hand and attempted to settle my deepest fears.

I have worked in a variety of medically complex situations over the course of my career, but it hits you on another level when something affects the health and safety of your own child. After a week, Gia was transferred to the local Children's Hospital NICU where she began to undergo a litany of tests and procedures. She was examined by a myriad of medical experts who were all collectively perplexed by her condition. Sadly, 2 weeks after Gia's birth we were still no closer to having any answers of what was plaguing our little girl and were forced to return home feeling disheartened and completely frightened.

It was during our stay at the Children's Hospital where we first met our daughter's genetics doctor. The first interaction with him played out completely opposite than how I imagined it in my head. He kindly introduced himself, then just stood over Gia while she lay there in her NICU crib and watched her for what seemed like hours while not speaking a word. Gia's neurologist showed up shortly thereafter for his initial assessment. Both doctors just stared at her silently, which was unsettling for us to say the least. My husband and I examined their faces closely, trying to uncover any clue of what they were thinking as our emotions were on a perpetual roller coaster. The two doctors began talking to one another and I was frantically trying to memorize, translate, and understand every word they were saying. I felt

© Springer Nature Switzerland AG 2021
A. F. Schrooten, B. P. Markovitz, *Shared Struggles*,
https://doi.org/10.1007/978-3-030-68020-6_37

like my head was going to explode, desperately seeking some guidance from either one of them.

As they stood there over Gia, my heart was pounding so hard it hurt. I was scared and angry, but mostly I was anxious. I wanted an answer at that very moment or at a minimum, something to the effect of "don't worry, we have seen this before, it is most likely..." Instead though, both doctors gave us no answers and very little explanation. They too were baffled. Our neurologist left but our genetics doctor stayed. I feel like he looked up and saw our utter anguish. He attempted to ease our worries and explained the next step was to perform a larger genetic panel, a test which takes over 3 months to receive final results. I felt helpless and frustrated, and I was worried no one would be able to figure out what was wrong with our daughter.

The next several months were torture. We were navigating unchartered waters and were beaten down physically, emotionally, and psychologically. We brought Gia to countless doctors, therapists, and had a steady stream of medical professionals visit Gia at our home. Looking back, none of it made a difference in the first 3 months, it was all one big exercise in futility. Without a clear genetic diagnosis, we were chasing our tail and treating every single symptom while not understanding the true underlying condition. During this time, we had no clue what we were up against. Some doctors were trying to provide treatment as if she was a fully functional child. She was often misdiagnosed which would lead to chaos at subsequent doctor visits. Our world was spinning out of control.

Our days were long and grueling, but the nights much, much worse. My husband and I had to tag-team the nights. I would go to sleep earlier in the evening once our other two children went to sleep and my husband stayed up with Gia until I woke up to pump and feed her. We took turns like this for months. I often woke up to post-it-notes left next to my bedside with things written on them like "I thought she was going to die tonight," or "this is so bad, I can't watch this." Looking back, it was by far the worst time in our lives. We were so scared and we still knew nothing about what was causing all of these ailments for our little love.

The day we received the results of Gia's Whole Exome Genetic Sequencing was the day that would forever change us. My hands shook, my palms sweaty, tears in my eyes, and my heart beating uncontrollably. I opened the email and downloaded the attachment to see the words "Causative variants in disease genes associated with reported phenotype: KIF1A-related disorder." A wave of relief came over me that we finally had an answer, although unaware of exactly what that answer meant. We immediately began Googling "KIF1A" and hours later, my husband and I were both in full embrace sobbing over what we had learned. This disorder was extremely rare, highly degenerative, and no cure or treatment currently existed.

As we started reading the symptoms of this horrific disorder, there was consolation because Gia already exhibited several of the symptoms and we were confident we finally had a diagnosis. Peripheral neuropathy (the EMG report showed little to no sensory or motor in both Gia's extremities), epilepsy (the EEG test showed abnormality and we were told seizures were likely to happen at some point), hypotonia (check), ataxia (probably the reason Gia was having difficulty with feedings, rapid eye movements, check), intellectual disability (delays in development, check), optic nerve atrophy (could be why Gia was still not making eye contact, note: make appointment with ophthalmologist), and cerebellar atrophy. Any parent who would read any one of these symptoms related to their child would undoubtedly be distraught. Imagine not one, but all of these things being present in your child—it is unbearable. There was relief that we finally had a diagnosis, but it was short-lived. Now that the information was sinking in, the relief dissipated and I felt like any moment I would just collapse to the floor. But the worst part was yet to come.

I contacted Columbia University the day we received Gia's genetic test results because they are spearheading the medical research and cure for this extremely rare disorder. What we came to learn is the KIF1A genetic mutation spans a wide spectrum of severity. The timing of my conversation with Columbia could not have come at a worse time. It was the middle of the day and my husband was at work, I had zero privacy because my wonderful neighbor was stopping by almost hourly to check on me, feed me lunch, and graciously set up cleaners to stop by our house to ease some of the burden that we were feeling. Although I was overwhelmed by their generosity and thoughtfulness, I felt like I had nowhere to go, nowhere to process what the stranger on the phone was telling me about my sweet, little daughter. I had a small notebook in my hand and was feverishly writing everything she was telling me. Until my heart stopped when I heard there were other children who died before their first birthday and others who struggled through childhood with a wide range of ailments. Columbia confirmed our daughter's gene mutation variant was one of the most severe and informed me two other children with the same variant both died before they were 1-year old. I found myself apologizing to this woman because I could not control my emotions. It was difficult to get my words out, difficult to form a sentence, and unbearable to ask the questions that I desperately needed answers to. By researching the KIF1A website we knew our daughter would suffer through major setbacks and be challenged her entire life, but I felt like my world came to an end after talking with the staff at Columbia. A total stranger, who would soon become my expert when no one else could help, just informed me our little girl's future was grim and she might not even reach her first birthday. How could life get any worse for a parent?

Four days later, we walked into our genetic doctor's office to review the results of the genetic testing we had received. I remember wanting to cancel the visit altogether. I was an emotional disaster. I had the diagnosis and I had researched endlessly for the previous 96 hours. By the time our doctor sat down in his chair directly across from us, I had already become part of the KIF1A.ORG Facebook group, spoken to other families and had contacted Columbia University's Chung Laboratory and spoken to one of the lead research doctors about Gia's specific gene variant. I did not want to go sit in front of another doctor, especially since this time I knew I would not be able to control my emotions and I did not understand what he needed to tell us that I did not already know.

Part of me thought we would get there and he could offer us some kind of hope, or better, he would tell us all of this was wrong. Instead however, he calmly unbuttoned his white lab coat and quietly pulled out a bright colored, plastic chair and sat down across from us. I immediately detected a shift in his demeanor and his face transformed from that of a medical professional to that of a friend and parent. Without speaking a word, I could tell he felt the same sadness we felt, and it was especially genuine. He handed us a folder with literature and documents associated with KIF1A and then there was this pause, this unnerving moment of silence. I did not know what he was going to say, and then I heard him take a deep breath and calmly he said, "I'm sure you know all of this by now, but can I offer you advice?" My husband and I looked at one another, tears already streaming down our faces and we both nodded "yes."

For the next hour, he gave us deep and compelling insight into his personal life and explained the story of how he lost his son. He explained the varying levels of grief that he and his wife experienced and how they independently and collaboratively coped with the tragedy. He explained his life after his son's tragedy and how he continued to work and would put this face on during the day, to get through what he needed to get through. He would then get home and need silence in order to process his feelings. His wife was the opposite, she was home during the day and the minute her husband came home, she needed to unload her feelings. He correlated his experience to our personal situations and at one point I smiled, realizing how similar he was to my husband and how similar I was to his wife. I felt the love he had for his son and the pain that he still was enduring. He went on to tell us to not forget about our other children. He explained how easy it will be to get lost in Gia's care and her unrelenting needs, but cautioned that our other children, albeit slightly different, have the same level of needs, maybe even more. He provided us invaluable advice about taking care of our marriage, making time for one another while ensuring we listen and recognize each other's varying methods of coping. He shared with us the alarming statistic of divorce in couples who lose a child. He stressed the importance of date nights and taking moments during the day to make sure we acknowledged each other in the stress of everyday life. He emphasized the importance of making sure our other two children knew that each day we were there for them just as much as we were for Gia. Not only was his advice compelling and moving, but the manner in which he communicated with us helped calm us and allowed us to see the significance and totality of our situation.

I believe fate brought this doctor into our lives. He knew walking into the appointment that day he would be delivering the worst news any parent ever wants to hear. He was the only one who could have related to our specific situation in the way he did, and he delivered a profound message which ultimately has helped guide us through our difficult journey. He did not lecture us, he did not talk over us, he sat and made us feel included in the discussion. He knew that at some point we would lose our beautiful daughter, he invited us into this club that no one ever wants to be a part of, and he guided us with love and care. We all cried together at that appointment and through our shared camaraderie we left the appointment feeling a sense of hope that we would be able to navigate the storm on the horizon. At the end of our meeting, I joked "maybe we should go out for dinner with you and your wife." It took him a moment but then he said, "you know what, I would like that." He then offered to see us in a year specifically saying, "I want to see you and see how YOU are doing."

The thing about living in our new rare disease world is that it is so lonely. People often do not know what to say or what to do and so they say nothing. It is also so very exhausting, and when coupled with our very busy lives, we are thrust into survival mode daily. I find myself constantly asking myself things like, how many seizures did she have today, how long were they, what did they look like, did they seem different, is this new medication working, is she in pain, did she do enough therapy today, why is the pharmacy not covering this med anymore, are we out of supplies … but mostly, does she feel our love?

Although we never met up for that dinner, I often think about reaching out to our genetics doctor and seeing him again. The meeting we had with him is a day that will never leave my memory. He taught us so much in the short hour we spent with him. He taught us how to get through this challenging time and how to steer our family in the most positive direction. He taught us to treat each day with Gia like it may be our last. He taught us to respect and nurture our marriage. But most of all, he gave us the courage and confidence that we would need to survive this, together.

Parent Commentary

What a gift this physician was for these parents. Rare is the physician who can sit across from a parent and tell them their child has a disease that will take their life and have a true understanding of what the pain of hearing those words feels like. Certainly, it does not take a physician who has experienced the loss of their own child to have empathy and compassion when delivering devastating news to a parent. However, there is an inexplicable bond that connects people who suffer a shared grief. This connection was immediately felt when Gia's parents recognized that this physician genuinely understood their anguish.

When a physician conveys information to us about our child and offers advice on how to move forward and live with the information (and many do offer this advice), we might think to ourselves—what does she know, she has not a clue what life will be like for me or my child. While we are always grateful for the physician who shows compassion and empathy, trusting their advice does not come easily when we know (or assume) they really do not understand what we are going through. If a physician wonders whether it is appropriate to share their personal shared experience with a parent, I would tell you that I believe the answer is "yes." It is appropriate and appreciated. The physician in this story could offer advice on topics that the majority of physicians do not have the personal experience to draw from—how their daughter's diagnosis would impact their marriage and their other children. Because this physician lived it, these parents trusted his advice and they clearly appreciated receiving it.

While I cannot speak for this physician because I do not know him, I do know that finding a way to use what we have learned through our own loss and grief to help others can help us in our own healing. As a geneticist, this physician cannot prevent parents from receiving a devastating diagnosis about their child; however, he can (and does) use his own experience to convey a grace and understanding that only a parent who has walked in their shoes can. And in doing so, I imagine that each opportunity he has to share his wisdom and understanding is an opportunity for him to heal his own grief just a little bit more. I hope one day that Gia's parents share that dinner with this physician and his wife. I suspect it will be a healing experience for all of them.

Physician Commentary

This is a truly inspirational story of a family finding a physician gifted in communication and empathy just when they needed it the most. This physician was able to truly offer meaningful advice in a holistic manner, not just medical recommendations. That this doctor had lost a son undoubtedly gave him more credibility with his advice, but this is a slippery slope and generalizing this experience is risky. For a physician to tell a family that because they too have experienced a tragic loss does not necessarily mean he or she "knows" what the family in front of them is experiencing and what they will go through. We all experience losses in life in a variety of forms. For any person, physicians notwithstanding, to empathize with any suggestion of the equality of loss (if such a measurement was even possible) and that the responses to losses of equal magnitude should be equal is presumptuous. This is one reason why we typically do not bring our own personal experiences into these difficult conversations.

This is why physicians are taught to never say: "I know what you are going through." Likewise, when asked by parents what we would do (about a medical decision) if we were in their place, our response should be: "I do not know. I cannot imagine what impact this situation would have on me and I don't want to pretend that I know."

This does not preclude physicians from offering advice, particularly when it comes to treatment options. We have the medical knowledge of the impact, success, and failure of the various options. But we should not presume we know how any given set of parents will feel or react in a unique situation.

This was a truly unique experience, and obviously this physician navigated this difficult situation very well. Perhaps what we really sealed this connection was not so much of this doctor's own loss, but rather of his empathy and ability to demonstrate his humanity.

The Life of the Party

38

A text page came from a close pediatric neurologist colleague, Daniel, who I also consider a friend.

"06: 05/09/14 11:10AM. Hey man. I have a challenge for you. Call me at 7-0904. No rush."

I saved the page in my pager, initially by happenstance, but I left it there because it eventually gained so much more meaning.

I am a Pediatric Physiatrist or a Pediatric Rehabilitation Physician or I practice Pediatric Physical Medicine and Rehabilitation. It is a mouthful. I am not sure that any of these names fit the job particularly well, but the concept is always the same: my role is to maximize function for my patients. They often have had a health change where there is a loss of function or they were born with a functional impairment. Or both. And that is where our patient comes in. I was about to learn more about myself and more about being a human on this earth than I had in any other context.

I called Daniel. He took a deep breath. He always does that when we start to talk about patients, but this was something else. It seemed to last forever. I imagined him exhaling large quantities of steam out of his nose on the other side of the phone. He did not speak. He took another deep breath. So I took a deep breath. It seemed like the right thing to do.

"Ok. Shoot." I blurted out, feeling plenty oxygenated at this point. He took another deep breath.

"I'm going to ask you to do something that I don't think you can do…" he said, trailing off at the end.

"It wouldn't be the first time." I snickered. He did not snicker. He took another deep breath.

"I just met this boy with an hourglass brain. It's new, or at least one side of it is. He has hemi CP and had a stroke on the other side. He's seven. There's not much brain left. We know what the textbooks say about this but this family is looking for hope. I'm looking to you to give it to them. I put a consult order in."

A. F. Schrooten, B. P. Markovitz, *Shared Struggles*,
https://doi.org/10.1007/978-3-030-68020-6_38

I can only imagine what that consult order in his medical chart could have said. In my head, I read "Hourglass brain. Please provide hope."

I took a look at his chart. His name is Jonathan. He was born in the early fall 7 years prior. There is small picture of him. He has wiry hair which is nearly the color of fresh snow and a complexion to match. He has more freckles than I can count, even on this postage stamp photo. His smile is crooked and it immediately tells a story. I can see every tooth in his mouth. His eyes are bright blue and the whites are fully exposed. It seems clear this kid knows how to party.

I scanned through the chart. It showed that he has a single ventricle in his heart instead of two. He was born this way. This chamber of the heart needs to pump to both the heart and the lungs and has to make sure that the right blood goes to the right places. It often involves multiple "plumbing"-type surgeries to sustain life. It frequently comes with complications. In this case, he had a large stroke around the time of birth on one side of his brain. He learned to walk around 15 months of age and made great use of his left arm and leg. His right-sided limbs were described in the chart as "helper hand" and "affected lower limb." He had weakness on this side, but there was movement there. Jonathan ran about in a fairly awkward fashion but certainly made it to his destination. He spoke in complete sentences. He needed extra help in school but he was learning.

This all changed 2 days before I met him when a clot formed in that single ventricle of his heart and travelled from his heart to the other side of his brain. He had a very similar stroke to that which he had around the time of birth, but this was on the other side. This is where the term, "hourglass brain" became poignant. When looking at an MRI of a brain in a common view, one would expect typical brain tissue to take an oval shape. I looked at pictures of Jonathan's brain and that common oval shape looked much more like the shape of an hourglass, with the majority of his brain tissue now damaged or completely gone due to injuries.

The majority of the brain structures necessary for movement, feeling, vision, talking, and thinking were either heavily damaged or absent. At that moment, I stopped looking at the MRI and chose to take my own advice. I find myself very regularly sharing with our medical students, residents, and fellows that one cannot let an MRI define the child. It may tell you what to look for, but children so frequently show you something different than what the MRI tells you. Jonathan was about to affirm that.

I stood up from my desk and headed toward his room on the cardiac unit. I took my favorite route, which goes outdoors for a while and has some shortcuts through some of the underground portions of the hospital. It is not a heavily travelled route, but there are many familiar faces of folks who are there daily. I try to gradually learn about their families and their interests. Maybe I will have something to bring into a patient room later. I arrived and found the door to Jonathan's room to be closed. I could not look in through the window, as it was plastered with pictures, art, and letters. It was an impressive collection for 2 days in the hospital and 1 day in this specific room. Taking a brief gaze into the room often allows me to go in more prepared. Sometimes I can catch a parent's eye so they know somebody is coming. That was not an option this time.

I knocked on the door and stepped in carefully. I looked to Jonathan first, as his name was on the door, though his mother caught my eye soon after. She was standing at the bedside and greeted me brightly with a warm "hello" and shook my hand.

"My name is Angela. It's nice to meet you. I've been told that I should look forward to meeting you." That was either Daniel's work or her strong social skills. I lean toward the latter.

"This is Jonathan," she said, communicating for him. This was a skill that she would develop to a much greater degree as the years went on.

We spoke about Jonathan. Angela was surprisingly buoyant for such a difficult context. Her eyes glowed, much like the boy in the postage stamp picture. Jonathan was laying in bed with his eyes partially open. His cheeks were round, red, and ruddy. On his body, he showed signs of a child who knew the insides of a hospital quite well. He had scattered scars and skin discolorations in locations where he could challenge his physicians to figure out how he got all these souvenirs from medical interventions. He had grown since that medical chart picture was taken. His mouth was open and it was clear that the tooth fairy had visited recently, and probably more than once. He was not moving much at all. His arms were held flexed at his body, legs straight as a board. He moaned every minute or so in a fairly coarse fashion. Each moan had similar pitch and cadence. It was a distinct moan. I would come to learn it well and hear it often from the hallways of this unit.

I spoke with Angela about the past 2 days and what has changed with Jonathan. This event happened abruptly. He was his typical self the day before. She described him as a boy with endless energy, one who could find enjoyment in nearly anything. He knew what he loved and he endlessly sought out that joy. He was the centerpiece of a blended family, with a number of older half siblings who adored him. We spoke about his love for certain Disney movies, for superheroes, and for our beloved local college football team. Angela held back tears as she shared this, clearly mourning the loss of function and fearing that this would persist.

She shared that he really was not moving either arm or leg much. He struggled to hold up his head. He was not looking around the room much, but "maybe he does sometimes," she said with a questioning tone. He really was not doing anything at all.

I examined Jonathan, paying close attention to how he interacted with me and his response to the environment. I gave him opportunities to move his limbs or follow commands or even withdraw to pain. There was no response. Angela cried quietly.

We spoke about recovery from stroke and about how it is often the job of the other side of the brain to help out when one side is injured. We spoke about how Jonathan did not have this option. Angela asked about recovery of movement, talking, walking, smiling, vision. I provided the most empathetic answer I could muster at that moment.

"I don't know."

I paused and took a long breath. Daniel's earlier hyperbolic-sounding breaths were now making much more sense to me. This was intense. I took another deep breath.

"What I can tell you is that there is a team of us here who aim to maximize Jonathan's joy. It is not fair for me to try to predict the future because I can't. But I feel like it is fair to aim our sights on Jonathan achieving joy."

Angela cried more, but these were a different kind of tears.

I could be easily and potentially rightfully criticized for saying those words at that time. How did I know that he could achieve joy, especially with such a large brain injury? He certainly did not seem to be doing so at the time. How could I give a mother such hope, if there was potential it would be false?

There is where medical science gets tossed to the side. There is plenty of art in physiatry that we so often struggle to quantify in medical journals. Philosophy creeps in as we discuss what is meaningful function and what is our purpose as a human. And this is where I lean on my mentors. It was an honor to train with a few of the greatest leaders in our field—those that could do the science but could also help to teach the humanity. They shared their patients with me—those families who trusted them more than any person on earth—and those patients were the reason why I could step out and make such a statement. Joy is a simple concept. When we boil it down, it can be something as simple as a familiar experience or the touch of a loved one. You know it when you see it. For some of these children, it is harder to find than for others.

We embarked on a journey with Jonathan that would span three more years. His therapy began. As a team, we worked on head control, trunk control, hand use, and communication. We worked hard to keep him awake during the day and ideally sleeping at night. He started to open his eyes more. Sometimes he would look about the room. Meanwhile, his heart challenged the rest of his body. His body was feeling the impact of a heart that struggled to suitably provide the blood that his organs needed. He spent more time in the hospital than out of the hospital, or at least that is how it seemed. Complication after complication occurred and nearly every organ system felt the impact. His vocal moan was a familiar one on that unit. We all learned to know it.

In terms of function as we commonly view it, Jonathan did not make progress. He did not gain full head control. He could not sit well. He did not use his hands or arms much. He did not stand or walk. I still have never heard him speak. We did not find an opportunity to bring him to our intensive rehabilitation unit as he just was not progressing in a practical enough fashion to feel that it would be helpful. But that is not Jonathan's story.

That bright-eyed fiery boy from the postage stamp picture did not disappear when he had his second stroke. We just needed to find a way to get it out. If my memory serves me correctly, the first glimmer of hope came when he passed gas. Angela told the story of it, sharing that he donned a huge smile immediately afterward and laughed. He passed gas again and his laugh got deeper. Desperate to see if this was real, Angela ran out and bought a whoopie cushion. It worked like a charm. Next came his favorite scene in the Disney Pixar movie, "Cars." He would consistently open his eyes and don that extra-large grin each time it came on. It was consistent and reproducible.

While Jonathan's medical chart depicted so much morbidity, pain, and complication, that was not the story in his patient room. This kid was a ball of joy. Jonathan developed an enormous fan club both in the hospital and out. Each admission came with stories of Jonathan's conquests while not in the hospital. He went to movies, returned to school, and became the centerpiece of his small town community. He found stability in his own complex, medically complicated, absolutely joyous way. He continued to celebrate each day in his own way as the seasons passed. He made it through another winter, only once getting admitted for a respiratory virus. Spring and summer passed and I did not see him or hear from family at all. He stayed out of the hospital and that was an achievement. But it did not last.

He was admitted once again in early Fall, just one week before his tenth birthday. Birthdays were a big deal for this boy. A superhero party was planned. The party location was moved to hospital, which was not going to keep anybody from enjoying it, especially Jonathan. I stopped by his room and peeked through a small space of visibility in the window. The look on Angela's face was unfamiliar. It lacked that buoyancy that I was used to seeing. The glow in her eyes was dulled. I entered the room and looked into Jonathan's eyes. He was not glowing much himself.

"I think the time has come," she shared. We spent many moments over the last 3 years touching on Jonathan's death, as it often seemed like he was close to dying, but also quite far away. But this time Angela had a feeling and she was right.

I could fill in the medical details that led to the end of Jonathan's life, but his story is not about medicine. This is about the party. It is a joy and honor to work in a place where superhero costumes are plentiful and easily located. After leaving his room that day, it took me less than 5 minutes to find a Captain America costume for myself and a Batman costume for Daniel. Jonathan's birthday was still more than 48 hours away. A time was set for the party. Invitations were sent out via email. Some of us briefly wondered if Jonathan would remain alive until his birthday. I subconsciously dreaded turning on my computer each morning at work, fearing that I would receive news that this party had to be cancelled for the wrong reasons. But he held on.

Daniel and I did our morning rounds, then donned our costumes and stopped by Jonathan's room. We had to wait to enter, as there was not enough room to fit all of the attendees. I could feel the excitement emitting through the closed door. We eventually entered the room to find the walls so full of birthday cards that paint was no longer visible. Angela had started to affix cards to the ceiling, given loss of surface area on vertical surfaces. Jonathan was, as always, the center of attention in the room. The physician in me briefly saw signs of life-threatening illness. I saw things that we all work so hard to prevent. But the human in me saw joy. I once again saw the light in his eyes. I saw the genuine smile on his face. This was a kid who was enjoying his last days as much as any other day. Jonathan partied hard for his birthday. He made it. He passed away the next day.

On the day Daniel paged me and took all of those deep breaths, neither of us knew how much this experience would change us as physicians and as humans. Jonathan took that hope that we instilled and thrived in a way that could not be imagined before it happened. I carry his inspiration with me each day when I meet children in new, difficult circumstances. And when parents ask me what to expect in the future, I humbly share that I recommend that we aim for joy.

Parent Commentary

The first thought that came to mind when I read this story is—*this doctor gets it*. He sees in his severely disabled patient what so many doctors fail to see. He sees a child who is not defined by his MRI. He sees a nonverbal child who can communicate. He sees a child who experiences joy despite all his limitations. He sees hope.

I also appreciate that when this doctor was asked by Jonathan's mother what his recovery from the second stroke would look like, he did not set out the worst-case scenario or make dire predictions about Jonathon's future. His seemingly simple statement of "I don't know" was hope-giving. He understands that the measure of joy and hope is unique for each patient and family.

I recognize that this doctor's perspective and focus of striving for joy despite the difficult circumstances his patients face has a lot to do with the specialty he practices. His job is to help his patients achieve their maximum potential within the limits of their disease or condition. While I do not know the make-up of his patient population, I would guess he has some patients where results are measured as an improvement in function and he has other patients where results are measured as "moments of joy," as he so poignantly shares.

Certainly, not every subspecialty lends itself to "finding joy" as its yardstick for success. Some specialists are tasked with fixing an issue that is capable of being fixed (surgeons), while others care for children who cannot be "fixed" in the way that many of us want (neurologists). Regardless of a doctor's particular specialty and measure of what constitutes a successful outcome, every doctor should be mindful to never extinguish hope or the possibility of joy. Hope and joy are always possible and can be nurtured in seemingly small ways, even as simple as donning a superhero costume to celebrate your dying patient's birthday.

Physician Commentary

I guess there is still "hope" for me as reading this story brought tears to my eyes. It is hard for physicians to accept "defeat," but our definition of defeat is often not the same as that of families and patients. Defeat to us (the opposite of hope) means not restoring a child to their prior state after an illness or injury. We aim to get them back to their baseline status, where the patient was before (usually measured by medical status, cognitive and physical functioning). If we cannot get the patient there, we often feel like we have lost, and some of us take it personally. That is what is so inspiring about this story, for although I do not practice physical medicine and rehabilitation, I am aware they set very concrete goals for functioning for their patient under treatment. For this physician who works in this space to find Jonathan's return to joy (without functional recovery) so meaningful, is awesome.

This story is a vibrant call for physicians to learn to recalibrate their goals when necessary. How often do we ask the families what they are hoping for? How often do we reset our goals to match theirs? Or to adjust our settings as the situation and families' goals change. Where this gets hard is that physicians must also do their best to set realistic expectations for families. Frankly, to simply say "I don't know" without providing at least a range of possible outcomes seems to be potentially shirking one's duty to inform. There are other ways and words to use that can provide hope and still give an appropriate estimate of prognosis.

Having said that, our ability to predict emotional or interactive recovery after illness and injury is probably well below our estimates of functional recovery, e.g., walking and talking. That is where this physician "stuck the landing," so to speak. Offering hope for finding joy is truly a nearly spiritual aspiration that you simply cannot take issue with. Too often physicians, with their strictly medical blinders on, do not look at the bigger picture. The picture does not get much bigger than joy.

Every Single Second Worth It

Paul was born in the middle of the night, at the beginning of Advent at one of the top Children's Hospitals in the world. With hints of his future red mop and an open sacral spine, Paul let out the sweetest, weakest cry and required immediate intubation. He and I were 90 minutes from home and our 1- and 4-year-old boys, my husband on the highway somewhere in between, all of us a world away from normal.

Later that day, as I sat by my babe post-op from his back closure, my mother's heart panicked: Paul's heart rate was high and climbing and he had a temperature. I had seen one of my children's pain management mishandled in the past and felt frantic not to let it happen again. Morphine please, and stat! No one seemed to move fast enough. What I did not realize at the time was that it would be "morphine, stat" for the rest of my boy's eight and a half years with us. Paul was suffering from severe dysautonomia due to Chiari II malformation. It would morph over the years and become much more manageable. But in the ICU, it presented as body afire and delirious, posturing, and at times flailing, heart racing, blood pressure through the roof, unable to gain weight while powering this furnace. He had calm periods as well, with sparkly eyes and an objectively beautiful face. But overwhelmingly, it presented as what it was: suffering.

At least as serious, this same brain stem malformation and compression was the reason Paul needed immediate intubation, not his 7-week prematurity as we hoped. Not only would Paul stop breathing, he would drop his oxygen saturations to zero in the space of seconds and need to be bagged back to pink—even though he was continuously ventilated. One of his primary nurses told me it was not something she had ever seen, even at this world-class NICU. His neurosurgeon, the top in his field for treating spina bifida, would later say much the same. My husband and I surely had never seen this, and, in part, my response was self-protective numbing. Even now, I cannot fully touch the pain of it.

I think it was Christmas night because both my husband and I were home with the boys, and I was receiving report over the phone from one of Paul's wonderful nurses. Part of a small team caring for him, she knew him well. She was telling me of all his desaturations that day and how serious and unique it was, how

© Springer Nature Switzerland AG 2021
A. F. Schrooten, B. P. Markovitz, *Shared Struggles*,
https://doi.org/10.1007/978-3-030-68020-6_39

inexplicable. I spoke so evenly with her, even laughing at points, that my husband looked at me when I got off the phone and said, without judgment, "I don't understand how you can laugh." I could not either. There is so much I could not understand.

The New Year brought Paul's third neurosurgery. The first two relieved his hydrocephalus and improved his breathing some, but at 4 weeks old, Paul was still severely desatting. This next surgery, a Chiari decompression of the cervical spine, was a risky surgery on a tiny baby with an immature vascular system. Though much less so in the hands of the top neurosurgical specialist in spina bifida in the country and the standard of care for symptomatic Chiari brainstem malformations, which as in Paul's case was life-threatening. But before we consented to this surgery, someone on the ICU team—I believe the APRN (advanced practice registered nurse) who headed the nursing team—was adamant that we meet with neurology. There were significant brain differences apparent on Paul's MRI scan, including a smaller than usual size. The young neurologist gently predicted Paul would never be independent and would likely die from one of his stop-breathing episodes. It was also possible Paul would one day be off the ventilator, no one could say.

"So he'll be our forever baby?"

"No, maybe more like an older toddler."

The neurologist himself was neutral and kind, with no apparent agenda other than to answer our questions. It seemed clear to me that the APRN believed this information might lead us to withhold surgery and by implication every further intervention, though no one said so explicitly. Looking back, I believe that at some level this registered with me and I tucked deep away the supposedly medically informed message: "Make sure his life is worth the effort. These are all extra extreme measures in the face of a dismal prognosis."

But the only thing that really made sense to us was that Paul's predicted vulnerabilities just meant he was all the more precious. Who throws jewels away just because they do not sing? Probably just as important were two other factors. First, we were familiar with this surgery as our older son had undergone it twice. Second, we were guided by our neurosurgeon who spoke kindly and forthrightly with us. He confirmed the risks, while humbly affirming his competence and success rate. He gently said that because "life with a ventilator is hard," but more so because Paul's current status was so life-threateningly unstable, that it was worth the comparably smaller risk to his life. He also made a simple but profound point to affirm our apparent unwavering commitment to Paul and spoke of finding me sleeping with full-blown mastitis with my head on Paul's bed. He spoke to our suffering and humanity, while lifting us up in his admiration. We had no hesitations and the family meeting later that afternoon went smoothly.

It was immediately after the family meeting that the head APRN made an explicit mention of ending care. Though she said nothing of it in front of the team, she pulled us aside before we left the room. Quietly and with tears in her eyes she said, "At some point you might want to ask, has he been through enough." I think I probably nodded.

"You know what I mean…?"

"Yes."

That was it. Such a small interaction, but it was like handing us an anvil as we were barely treading water in a moonless night. Though some notion that death might be better for Paul than a life of suffering was perhaps inevitable, never had we imagined it being of our hand or our decision.

When that surgery did not completely stop Paul's desatting episodes amid his continued suffering, this unfettered death idea—the heaviest of weights floated without context, without medical, moral, and psychological companionship as we wrapped our heads around what she was suggesting—plummeted us into a deep, distressing confusion.

It is three and a half weeks later and I am holding Paul, in the dark, propped on pillows like the prince that he is to accommodate the breathing and feeding tubes and wires. It is the night before his tracheostomy and G-tube surgeries. The general surgeon stands tall in front of me, explaining they will have to open my now 6-pound baby from chest to belly button instead of doing laparoscopic surgery because he might have a malrotated intestine. I sign the consent forms. And I wonder, is this the stuff we are not supposed to do? Since the APRN's comment, the voices in my head (and nightmares as I sleep) began speaking of doing more harm than good—and of being simultaneously unable to stop Paul's suffering and unable to care for my other children. But we have no guidance on what that might mean or with whom we should speak.

I begin to panic. But I cannot move to find someone to talk to—I do not have help moving Paul from my lap and the tubes are literally forbidding. It is not the first or last time that the impulse to act on my dark panic will be stayed—not guided by ethical discussions or medical experience—but by some other hand. The next morning they cut a hole in Paul's larynx and place his first trach.

Though we followed the inevitable tide toward and through Paul's trach and G-tube surgery, the lead up and aftermath were indeed dark and difficult. We tried very hard to understand the ramifications of ventilatory support in the context of suffering and a body that seemed wired to not live. But we were almost entirely alone.

I do not remember exactly who we spoke to about what it would mean to move Paul to comfort care or even whether we knew it was comfort care or hospice or just waiting to withdraw support. If we ended interventions, did that mean *future* dangerous and invasive surgeries? Or did that mean ventilatory support itself? What about a tracheostomy—an invasive surgery meant to connect him to the vent—why were we consenting to this? How about the open surgery to place a G-tube? We did not know who to ask, how to ask, or what we were even asking.

As this darkness enveloped us, the team spoke with two voices. On the one side, each progressive standard-of-care intervention was spoken of as inevitable and supportable. On the other was the APRN, insisting on our meeting with neurology, her comments, and her push that we speak with the palliative care team (a conversation which clarified so little I remember nothing of it.)

We spoke to the Catholic chaplain who, based on what we told him, told us we could withdraw care. But if you are drowning in foreign medical concepts and technologies and prognoses, how do you accurately represent your child's case for such discernment? We spoke to our families, who with a full and absolute commitment to us and our children, to life, and the vulnerable, did not understand any more than we did about what counted as "extreme measures" and what counted as standard of care—who indeed trusted our own representation of the information, knowing our commitment to the same standard of ethics. We sought out other families who had faced this difficulty, but though we found a couple of families with somewhat similar stories, none faced what we did in terms of degree of apnea or of autonomic suffering.

Where were the skilled medical staff? Where were the folks with experience with trachs and vents, with knowledge of the basic ethics of technological medical support, and with a commitment to each patient's life regardless of his or her unrelated cognitive or physical disabilities?

I cannot overestimate the nightmare of this confusion.

In the last couple of weeks of Paul's stay at his first hospital, I ask his nurse whether she thinks we can do this. We are blanketing Paul when his temperature drops, then removing the blankets when his temperature rises, over and over, a simple and calm variation of Paul's often terrible instability. She reiterated the support we would have from homecare nursing and said further, "Yes it will be hard. But anything worth doing is hard." That is the kind of thing you tell a family.

The day we transferred to our local hospital, a month after Paul's trach surgery, things were as murky as ever. Except now we were leaving whatever ballast we did have in the comfort of the nurses and doctors who loved Paul and were plunged into completely unknown waters. I remember feeling so dizzily confused. What had we even decided? Why were we transferring? If his case was hopeless and if the ventilator was keeping him alive only for our own comfort and not his, was the plan to train to take him home or to prepare to allow his body to decide without "extreme" supports? Given all of this, who were we going to be to this new team? What were we asking of them? Would they help us navigate?

To the end of our stay at the first NICU, the APRN emphasized that the terminology we should be using was "comfort measures only." Was urinary catheterization a comfort measure? Antibiotics for UTI? Increased O2? What fell into what category and on what basis?

This vague idea of comfort care coupled with a very real DNR (the only thing we agreed to for sure was that we did not want them to break Paul's ribs with chest resuscitation) had a significant impact on the care he received at the local ICU. It is too much to document here, but as an apparently disposable patient, this rare and utterly unstable child would be cared for by a revolving door of nurses and intensivists, almost none of whom committed to understanding him. Thus, while his suffering worsened and his stay at the new hospital was wrongly and hopelessly predicted to be more than a year versus the 4 weeks we had been told, our despondency deepened to despair.

By grace, this bottoming out resulted in a full rejection of a DNR and palliative care only, and an explosive demand for continuity of care and treatment for his dysautonomia. A pure gift, Paul lit up our lives for eight and a half years, every single second worth it.

As of this writing, it has been 10 years since my family walked this path. And it has been only in writing this that my husband and I have worked through what we think should or should not have happened and why. Here is our family's perspective and what we ask physicians to consider.

First, as a medical professional, please know that your voice has an outsized effect. You represent authority and experience—all the more so the more complicated the case is—and the assumption is that you have worked through these issues far more than patients and their families have. In this context, there is no such thing as an ethical sidebar. Whatever you say opens doors to possibilities, fears, and altered conceptualizations—especially for families in crisis. Furthermore, if you have something to say of this magnitude, you must say it in front of your peers. If you have to whisper it, it is probably not licit.

Second, any major suggestion you make to a family must be backed up with resources to support the decision-making process. This includes an explicit and thought-out ethical basis.

On that note: third, there is no ethical basis for suggesting that treatment, lifesaving or otherwise, be withheld from a child because they have or are predicted to have cognitive and/or physical disabilities. This is ableism and it is inhumane.

Treatments—assuming they are available and inherently licit, and certainly if they are standard of care—should only be withheld if the specific conditions they are intended to treat have a terminal prognosis and the treatment would at best prolong life but at a cost to the patient. In Paul's case there was no definitive prognosis and, predictions aside, the neurologists and neurosurgeon agreed it was possible he would outgrow his apnea. And he did, eventually spending large chunks of time off the ventilator.

Furthermore, treatments—especially those that are foreign and overwhelming to patients, like the short-term oscillator and the long-term ventilator—and the ethics that undergird their use, should be well understood by all medical staff. There should be a plan in place to allow families to become similarly familiar with them so that their appearance of being "extreme measures" can be contextualized. For treatments that will be continued at home, this would include contact with families further on their journey with these technologies.

Without this context and these data points, drastic decision-making about these treatment modalities cannot be considered informed. If we were again to have a child in Paul's situation, we would not consider home ventilation to be any more "extreme" than wheelchairs or insulin pumps.

Fourth, and this is very important: Suggesting that treatments may be withheld because a child is disabled is to tell parents that their child's life is less worth saving. There really is no neutrality here and passing these suggestions off as "allowing parents to decide" is at best a cop out. Coming from anyone, such suggestions are a violence to a family's well-being. Coming from a medical professional, again with your larger impact, so much more so.

Finally, there are no backdoor escapes from suffering in this life, though we all seek exactly these outs. I don't know what it is like to watch countless children and their families suffer, only my own and my friends. But I do know what it is like to have a counterbalance to that suffering, something I can only guess is woefully inaccessible in an ICU: the times in between crises, the kind of joy that only comes from enduring suffering, the depth of friendship with fellow caretakers, and the love that finds in brokenness an unspeakable preciousness.

You may not have a holistic handle on what families are dealing with in the ICU and beyond. However, you do have access to these families before they themselves might be able to see these gifts. Be so very careful not to tip the scale in favor of fear and nihilism; this is not mercy, it is theft.

Instead, like the nurses I mentioned and the neurosurgeon—speak, yes with honesty, but always with encouragement and love. If there is an obstacle that brings you to your limits—as Paul's dysautonomia and apnea did for so many of us—*fight*. Fight for a solution. Fight for hope—whatever that hope looks like. If the same effort that went into trying to get us to stop treatment had gone into researching treatment for dysautonomia and to help his apnea, Paul would have received relief months sooner.

We fully understand and have experienced times when there is no hope except for peace in letting go, even unto death, as we accept that treatments would only do harm. However, not every "extreme" measure falls into this category. Not every "extreme" measure is optional, no matter how foreign it may be to new families. In these cases, the physician's job is not to help families determine whether licit, helpful standard-of-care treatment may be withheld: it is modeling the bravery and providing the knowledge needed to swim through the dark waters toward the shores of a new normal.

Parent Commentary

There are so many important messages imparted in this story that have been so beautifully and painfully shared by this parent. It is heartbreaking to hear how abandoned this family felt by the medical team during a time when they so desperately needed guidance. In all honesty, I do not know how or who provides the level of support and guidance parents need when faced with the many difficult decisions this family faced. However, I wholeheartedly agree with the summary of points made in the conclusion of this story. It cannot be stressed enough that a child's cognitive and/or physical disability and technology dependence is not determinative of quality of life and should never be the sole basis for life-altering decision-making. Nor, do I believe, should guidance for decisions regarding intervention come only from people who never see our children outside of the hospital setting.

It sounds like Paul spent the majority, if not all, of his hospital time in the intensive care unit and that the primary teams involved in his care were the ICU teams and neurosurgery. I can understand how it might not be within the purview of these particular teams to provide the information and resources this family needed beyond the immediate needs of their son. However, given that they must regularly see patients with the level of involvement Paul had, I think it is reasonable to expect them to connect Paul's parents with the people who could collaborate with these specialty teams to provide the support and resources Paul's parents needed to navigate their path forward. The people who come to mind for me are the palliative care team, and in this case it sounds like palliative care was asked to consult. Unfortunately, Paul's mother did not find them to be helpful.

When I read that Paul's parents rejected "a DNR and palliative care only" and instead demanded "continuity of care and treatment for his dysautonomia," I thought: if only their experience with the palliative care team had been a positive experience, they might have had the advocate they needed to ensure their values and goals for Paul were honored and respected when faced with treatment decisions. It did not have to be palliative care *or* treatment; it could have been both.

Palliative care is a relatively new subspecialty and is not well understood by parents or even doctors. When my son was discharged from the hospital on a ventilator over 20 years ago, there was no such thing as a palliative care team. When he was 14 years old and we were deciding whether to bring the palliative care team on board, I was initially resistant to the idea because I thought palliative care was end-of-life care. However, I now understand that palliative care is not the same as hospice care. Palliative care is complementary to, not in lieu of, other therapies and treatments for our child's condition or disease.

Paul's mother presents a comprehensive picture of the world parents are abruptly thrust into when their child is born with a complex and potentially life-ending condition. The decisions that have to be made are overwhelming and parents desperately need guidance and support from the experts caring for their child. I recognize that there is no simple solution for providing parents with the extraordinary level of support they need, but the points offered by Paul's mother should be given great weight. I also believe, notwithstanding their disappointment to Paul's parents in this story, that having the support of a qualified palliative care team as soon as it is known that the child has a life-limiting condition can be a valuable resource for parents. However, and as has been stressed in other stories in this book, to be successful, it is imperative that parents understand that palliative care does not mean hospice care and that their child can and will (if it is what the parents want) receive ongoing and aggressive treatment for acute and chronic issues while on palliative care.

Physician Commentary

There are almost too many lessons to list in this story and advice to physicians from this family. I will comment on a few aspects. First, this family does not sound like they received the support they needed at a critical time. At least when it came time to plan for chronic ventilatory support. This is not the domain of intensive care physicians or neurosurgeons. In most pediatric programs, it is the pulmonary team who guide children and families on the path of home mechanical ventilation. This multidisciplinary group of physicians, nurses, advanced practice providers, and respiratory care practitioners is invaluable in helping families understand the scope of what this commitment means and helps them every step of the way. In my opinion, offering home mechanical ventilation without this team is like offering neurosurgery without the input of the neurosurgeon.

Palliative care today is decidedly not the same as hospice or end-of-life care. Modern palliative care teams are uniquely qualified to help families cope with complex diseases, weigh risks and burdens, ease discomfort, and more, all the while distinctly incorporating the values and goals of each family as distinct from every other. Palliative care does not bring any agendas to these situations. They listen, listen, and listen more. They get to know parents and children sometimes better than any other care team. If a family is a small flock, palliative care teams function as shepherds, calmly, wisely, and compassionately guiding, based upon the family's values, not their own. If we had unlimited resources, palliative care should be involved with every child who has three or more consulting services and an uncertain future. Actually, I made these criteria up just now, but the point I hope is well taken. Do not wait until you are at wit's end, confused, and uncertain about how to manage such extreme complexity. Ask for and welcome this team's support.

Finally, I want to remind our readers that at least in the United States, parents are regarded as the surrogate decision-makers for their children who are either too young to make decisions for themselves or cognitively unable to do so. The premiere principle in medical ethics today in our society today is autonomy. The patient alone has the authority to determine what is to happen to their body. Although even this pillar of a principle has limits (technically, suicide is illegal), it is still the bedrock of decisions in American medicine. Many adults, when asked the question, "do you want to be mechanically supported for breathing and feeding if you have no meaningful chance of recovery?", answer in the negative. Parents must answer questions like these as their child's surrogate decision-maker; what they believe their child would want. Of course, there is probably never any way to actually know; adults may share answers to such questions with each other and record them in the form of advanced directives. My point is that we must always be looking out for the child's best interest, which may or may not align with what the parent wants. Frankly, I do not have an answer as to how to operationalize this in a definitive manner. The best one can do is put yourself in the child's shoes. What would I want for myself in this situation?

Why do I bring this up in relation to this story? Because offering limitation of care to a child who is likely to never walk or talk, or who may spend their entire life dependent on machines to sustain their breathing and nutrition, is absolutely an ethical mandate for physicians. Insisting on such limitation is wrong, but offering it is right. It is what a consenting adult would want as a choice. Children should have that option as well.

Partners in Hope

40

As a pediatric palliative care consultant and a pediatric intensivist, most of my patients have complicated medical conditions. I learn a great deal from each of them and from their families, but one patient in particular pushed me to grow as a physician and a human being.

Nathan is a 3-year-old boy with Gaucher disease type 2. Gaucher disease is a lysosomal storage disorder, which means that because a certain enzyme is missing, fatty chemicals build up in the body, including the liver, spleen, and bone marrow. Gaucher type 2 is a very rare, rapidly progressive form of the disorder which affects the brain as well as other organs in the body. Children with Gaucher type 2 usually develop neurologic symptoms around 3–6 months of age, such as poor development, seizures, abnormal movements, and difficult swallowing, and most children die before the age of 2.

When I met Nathan, he had already undergone an experimental stem cell transplant to provide him with cells that made that important enzyme. His parents had searched the world over and traveled extensively in order to find any treatment that held out some hope of cure or even improved quality of life. Nathan had made it through some pretty scary times during his transplant, but he had survived to discharge and they had been enjoying their time at home.

Nathan was able to eat by mouth and often smiled. He loved hearing music and watching his mom dance. But several months before his admission to my hospital, he started having seizures and abnormal movements. When the movements got worse, his parents brought him in for evaluation. That was the start of what ended up being a two and half month hospitalization, most of which was in the Pediatric Intensive Care Unit (PICU). During this time, he had what seemed like constantly shifting patterns of abnormal movements which took a tremendous toll on his little body. He also had a prolonged course of respiratory failure requiring intubation and mechanical ventilation. Eventually he was able to be extubated, but he continued to require support for his breathing, ranging from simple oxygen to noninvasive positive pressure through a mask.

© Springer Nature Switzerland AG 2021
A. F. Schrooten, B. P. Markovitz, *Shared Struggles*,
https://doi.org/10.1007/978-3-030-68020-6_40

The day I met Nathan and his parents, I had been forewarned that it was "not a good day." Nathan's mom and dad were both exhausted and worried about their son. They were also extremely frustrated that his abnormal movements and increasing difficulty breathing were being attributed by the medical teams to the progression of his disease. Because Nathan had a successful transplant, his body now made the enzyme that is missing for kids with Gaucher disease. His parents wanted us to look for other reasons for his symptoms. They also wanted us to make him feel better. Most of all, they wanted us to believe in their son the way that they did.

I will never forget the way that Nathan's mother described her commitment.

"I know what the statistics are for Gaucher type 2," she said, "but I also know my son. And my mama's heart tells me there has to be something more for him and I am not going to stop until I find it. I can't give up on this kid," she continued. "I mean, look at him!"

She often shared pictures with me that captured Nathan's best moments—the smiles, the times when he made eye contact with her, and the special connection they had together. Occasionally I got to witness those moments too, though I also witnessed many moments when Nathan was clearly suffering.

Unfortunately, in the first few weeks of his hospital stay, many providers only saw the bad moments, causing them to focus on the injustice of Nathan's extended suffering and wonder whether ongoing aggressive care was ethical. Others did not think that Nathan had much awareness of his environment, attributing his occasional smiles to facial reflexes. However, the time I spent in his room watching him and talking with his parents allowed me to know differently. It also helped me to see Nathan as they saw him, as a beautiful, brave little boy fighting a terrible disease.

As the weeks went by, I took care of Nathan as his palliative care consultant and then as his PICU doctor and then back again. We worked with neurology to try to develop a logical plan to decrease his abnormal movements, but there was really no evidence upon which to base our plan. Everything we did was extrapolated from other types of movement disorders or even from the anecdotal experience of individual providers who had small cohorts of patients with disorders similar to Gaucher.

At Nathan's parents request, we conferenced regularly with the neurodevelopmental specialist who had overseen his stem cell transplant. When one medication did not work, we tried another, always cautiously and with some trepidation because pretty much every drug that is used to treat movement disorders decreases muscle tone, and Nathan was already dangerously weak. Throughout this course, Nathan's parents were indispensable members of the team. They kept meticulous track of his reaction to different medications and how the varying patterns of his movements responded. And they never let us stop striving to make things better.

The day that Nathan left the hospital was a special celebration. To be clear, Nathan was not "fixed"; in fact, he was still incredibly fragile. He still had nearly constant movements whenever he was awake, but the movements were less intense, less debilitating, and did not threaten his breathing the way they once had. His oxygen levels were staying in normal range almost all the time, with constant monitoring, a range of support from mask ventilation to nasal cannula, regular treatments to help keep his airways clear, and frequent suctioning to clear his secretions. He was tolerating feedings through his gastrostomy tube. His parents were nervous about providing all the care he would need at home but ecstatic about finally getting out of the hospital. They thanked me for being a part of Nathan's team, for listening to them, and for believing in Nathan. They expressed gratitude to all the PICU staff. But their highest admiration was for their son. "We are so proud of this little guy," they beamed. "He did it! We knew you could do it, Nathan!"

It is difficult to articulate all the lessons I learned through caring for Nathan and his parents. But the main one is this: physicians are taught to practice evidence-based medicine and to work only within their own realm of expertise. When no practice guidelines exist and the only evidence is tangentially related at best, I learned that there is value in being willing to step outside my professional comfort zone to partner with a family.

Nathan's parents had already risked everything—their jobs, finances, personal health, and other relationships—to help their son have the best life he could. Could not I risk a little too? Could not I embrace a little inconvenience and swallow a little pride to reach out to physicians in distant hospitals and read Facebook testimonials and texts by other parents in order to find and critically evaluate every last possible option to improve Nathan's care? That was what his parents asked for, and, to their credit, it really was exactly the kind of care Nathan deserved.

In the months since Nathan left my hospital, he has sustained several further setbacks. After a prolonged respiratory illness, he eventually received a tracheostomy. His weakness and movement disorder do seem to be progressing and a recent MRI confirmed significant loss of brain volume. He has received most of his care at another hospital closer to their home, so I have not seen him in quite some time, but I spoke with his father recently by phone. He sounded tired and sad as he talked about their struggles to come to terms with Nathan's decline. I told him how sorry I was, that I wished things could be different. It is a strange mind-space to know what is likely to happen and to simultaneously, wholeheartedly hope and strive for something different.

Parents of children with life-limiting medical conditions are forced to inhabit this space; they know too well the oscillation between optimism and despair, visualizing the dream and being confronted by the reality. Being a physician for these children and their parents requires sensitivity to that experience and, I believe, a willingness to genuinely align oneself with the parents' hope. Only by doing so does one earn the right to speak the painful truth, to gently help them prepare for the loss to come. It is, I am discovering, the greatest art of palliative care or of good medicine in general. Being a part of Nathan's journey drove home that lesson for me and it continues to be confirmed in different ways by each child and family I care for. These are humbling lessons to be sure, but I am immensely grateful to have the opportunity to learn them.

Parent Commentary

All parents have hopes and dreams for their children. For the parent of a child with a life-limiting condition, hope is a powerful thing. It is what drives us, carries us, and comforts us in the darkest of times. We have seen our child overcome insurmountable odds despite being told by medical professionals that our child is going to die or is not going to progress beyond the fragile state they are in at that time.

We know more about our child's disease than most physicians possibly can because we only have our child to focus on. We have done our research and read every book and article we can find on our child's condition. We communicate with other parents all across the globe whose children live with the same disorder as our child and whose children are cared for by the top specialists in their child's disorder. When our child's doctors do not have the answers, we reach out to our vast network for information and guidance. Most importantly, we know our child. We understand our child's body language, facial expressions, and reactions. Our child's eyes can convey more information than any monitor or test can.

It is a delicate balance to live with the knowledge of our child's disease and prognosis, our child's present condition, and still have hope that tomorrow can be a better day. A parent who lives with the hope of a better tomorrow for their child is not a parent who refuses to accept the reality of their child's disease and prognosis. Hope is how we survive. Hope is what gives us the strength to get up each day, put one foot in front of the other, and be the best caregiver, advocate, and voice for our child that we can be. We recognize that the day will come when we will have to say "enough." But until that day, we hope.

Nathan's physician listened to his parents and trusted their knowledge, experience, and belief in their son. Even though she could not "fix" Nathan, her willingness to partner with Nathan's parents and step outside her professional comfort zone ultimately gave Nathan more good days. He was able to leave the hospital and be in the comfort of his own home and in the care of his loving family. It was what his parents had hoped for.

Nathan's physician honored his parents' hope, and by honoring their hope, she gave them strength. Strength to advocate for new and experimental treatments; strength to overcome their nervousness in taking Nathan home knowing the level of his care was greatly increased; strength to get up each day and provide the extreme caregiving Nathan required despite their overwhelming exhaustion. And in the face of Nathan's declining health, her compassion gave Nathan's parents strength to endure the tomorrow that might not be a better day.

Physician Commentary

As pediatricians, we like to believe we are "softer" with patients and families than doctors who care for adults. Children are cute and their diseases are not self-inflicted as are many adult diseases. We like to think we know how to communicate better and build rapport with children and their parents. In truth, we can be just the opposite at times. We can feel threatened by parents of children with complex conditions because they often come armed with literature, support group information, and stories of treatments that seemed to have worked on others. We think we are "evidence-based" and bedside scientists and only employ proven therapies, regarding anything out of the mainstream as "snake oil."

What this physician did with Nathan and his family was to recognize their commitment, try to see the child how they saw the child, and trust that thinking outside the box on innovative treatments was worth trying for Nathan. She truly partnered with them, and even if she did not believe in the child as the parents did, she believed in the parents.

There is another lesson here for physicians, particularly those who only work in inpatient settings. We see children with complex conditions come into the hospital only when they are ill and never get to see them as they are at home. A child who is critically on life support in the PICU who looks to us as unresponsive with a poor prognosis is not the child the family knows and loves. We must try to look at the child through the parents' eyes and truly understand that they are the only ones who could ever know and see the child as a complete (small) person and not just a sick baby. We must be constantly vigilant not to project our values on others. And we should never state what we would choose for a child if we were in the parents' shoes. No amount of intellect or knowledge can ever truly put us in the position of the parents in front of us unless we have experienced the same condition in our own children.

When I was in my pediatrics residency, parents used to ask me if I had children of my own. I did not and told them. They constantly reminded me that I could never understand how they feel until I had children of my own. At the time I did not appreciate the depth of the parent-child bond. Then I did have my own children and I understood right away that they were right all along.

Answers for Rosie

41

"Today is the day when I will finally get an answer," I tell myself as I am driving to the hospital to be admitted with Rosie for another EEG. Rosie was born a few weeks early after a seemingly normal pregnancy. At birth, she was found to have profound brain damage which was later revealed to have happened while she was inside my belly, unbeknownst to me. She has already endured a month long NICU stay, countless IV pokes, two spinal taps, multiple ultrasounds and MRIs, and G-tube surgery. Rosie has earned many NICU Beads of Courage. What should have been a normal second baby postpartum period became a life upended in a blur of sleeplessness, pumping breast milk, first baby toddler tantrums, and an eventual move across the country to obtain better healthcare for Rosie. Our NICU stay was full of both good and bad interactions with doctors and healthcare staff, which made us into hospital veterans and made me ready to fight for an answer for my girl.

Rosie has endured EEGs before, first in the NICU for 5 days when we were told she had "very little brain activity." Then three more times at our local Children's Hospital when we were told her "background looked awful" but there was nothing they could do about that. We have been repeatedly dismissed by our neurologist, who is a neonatal epilepsy specialist. He advised us that "her brain is already significantly damaged, so having seizures is not really going to do anything worse." He does not know that her name is Rosie and he cannot remember my name either.

I have known something is wrong with Rosie's movements for over 8 weeks now. As a physician myself, I suspect she has infantile spasms, a poorly understood form of epilepsy often associated with brain damage that kids like her have. I religiously recorded videos. I emailed them to her neurologist and was told "who knows, do another EEG." I have connected with other parents who have been unequivocal in their, admittedly, Internet diagnosis. But no answers have come for Rosie. No treatment options have been proposed and no hope for her future has been offered. I feel I must seek a second opinion elsewhere.

This time, the EEG will be 24 hours or more. As the EEG tech sets up Rosie's study, I notice again the scars on her chin and forehead from the NICU—the metal EEG leads left on so long they eroded her delicate baby skin. I know this night will

© Springer Nature Switzerland AG 2021   223
A. F. Schrooten, B. P. Markovitz, *Shared Struggles*,
https://doi.org/10.1007/978-3-030-68020-6_41

be the next of many more to come in a hospital together. Throughout the evening, Rosie does the strange movement in several clusters which are recorded on the EEG. I try, but fail, to make sense of all the squiggly lines going past on the monitor. I cannot sleep for the anxiety of a possibly devastating diagnosis to come in the morning.

When the neurology team comes to round in the morning, they have reviewed her study as a team. I am so reassured by having the opinion of multiple doctors. The head neurologist visits us personally. He looks at me, then at Rosie, and says, "I think it is unethical not to treat your daughter's seizures." I slowly release the breath I did not realize I had been holding in.

He takes time with us, he looks into our eyes when he talks, he touches Rosie's hand, and he makes her smile. I am relieved that someone is finally making an effort to make a good decision for my child. But I also feel sick to my stomach knowing that Rose was suffering while not being treated over the past several months and sad that the first neurologist had become so jaded he could not even consider my input as a parent. While the news of a diagnosis of infantile spasms is difficult, I finally feel like everything will be okay because someone has actually listened to me. Someone has actually taken the time to treat my daughter as a human being and not as a laundry list of diagnoses and a horrendous MRI image.

He was not in the room for more than 10 minutes, but he gave us all of those 10 minutes without checking his phone or dismissing my questions to plow over me with his prejudgmental thoughts. We are two people talking to each other about a very small person's well-being with a combined common goal.

The weeks that follow of ACTH treatment are difficult. The medication takes 5 days to ship to our house and the cost is over $30,000. We are assisted with the cost and taught how to administer the shots. Rosie is kept in the hospital until the medication is delivered to our house due to the seriousness of the diagnosis. I have to inject my daughter twice a day with a strong medication that makes her hungry, irritable, and sleepless. Rosie starts to get better. She starts to eat very well, something she has not consistently done since birth. She finally gains weight, and, as we taper off the medication, she returns to her happy, spasm-free self. But the demon of the spasms returning is always hovering over our heads and I am unable to bring myself to throw out the tiny amount of medication we have left in our fridge, probably worth $200 or more. Seeing it there next to her bottles of milk is like a talisman against evil.

When we see the neurologist at our follow-up appointment, he takes the time to go through the entire EEG video with me. He shows me the squiggly lines that are important along with the part of the video which shows particular movements that concern him. I can now understand better what to look for and advocate for my girl. He spends over an hour with us. We are not just another box to tick off on his schedule. He holds Rosie's hand and says "little Rosie, you are looking so good" and he genuinely cares that she is. He is interested in his job, in the science of neurology, and in his patients. We continue to see him every few months and Rosie finally starts to progress in her development.

I know that we have many more battles to fight as we move forward. It is a constant battle not to give into the rhetoric we were told on a regular basis by several health professionals—that Rosie will never walk, talk, eat, or go to school. That Rosie is nothing. However, with this new team and, most importantly, with a neurologist who believes my child deserves a chance at living her best life possible, I feel reassured that while things will not be perfect, they will be okay. Rosie will go to school and she may talk with the aid of a communication device and she may walk with the aid of equipment. And above all, we cannot know the capacity of the human brain no matter how damaged and we can never underestimate the power of simple kindness and hope.

Parent Commentary

Parents of children with a devastating diagnosis always want some idea of what to expect for their child's future. But we also want to have hope. A physician can offer an opinion based on their experience and the data and literature available. However, no two patients are exactly the same and every prognosis given to a parent should include, "but every child is different."

The first neurologist offered no treatment—or hope—for Rosie based on a picture of her brain. One of the first things I was told as the parent of a technology-dependent child is to "look at the child, not the numbers." The same can be said in the context of making a prognosis: look at the child, not the scan.

Compassion and hope are closely intertwined. The second neurologist displayed compassion by giving Rosie's mother his time and undivided attention, by offering a treatment option for Rosie and through his interactions with Rosie. He saw in Rosie a child who smiled. A child's smile alone is reason enough to have hope. This physician's compassion translated to "my child matters" to Rosie's mother. His compassion gave Rosie's mother hope. Not unrealistic hope, but the kind of hope a parent needs to get up each day and keep on keeping on. Hope that allowed Rosie's mother to envision a future of possibilities for Rosie and to believe that Rosie could have a good life despite her diagnosis.

When your child has a disease or condition that will significantly impact them their entire life, the future feels ominous and overwhelming. Hope is essential. A physician may be reluctant to consider treatment options or suggest anything other than the worst-case scenario because they do not want to get a parent's hopes up. However, hope is not fixed in time. It evolves and changes as our child gets older and we come to have a better understanding and acceptance of our child's condition and its impact on their life. Physicians do not need to task themselves with tempering a parent's hope, because there is a worse thing than false hope—it is no hope.

Physician Commentary

Giving a prognosis—predicting the course of a condition—is one of the most important facets of being a physician. There are some conditions where the prognosis is highly predictable and accurate. The most extreme example is brain death (or death by neurologic criteria). After being declared brain dead, after a series of meticulously performed examinations meeting national guidelines, no one—ever— has woken up. This diagnosis has a 100% accuracy prediction rate. However, particularly when it comes to children whose brains are continually developing (or are supposed to do so), our ability (and I am not a pediatric neurologist but work with them almost daily) to predict the future after damage is limited. The best we can hope to do is offer a range of possible outcomes. I myself cringe inside when I hear physicians providing absolutes about prognosis.

But there is another side to this and similar situations that likely guides some physicians' attitudes. Many have had parents (a minority but vocal set) come back to them years after taking care of a "neurologically devastated" child who state (paraphrased): you never told me how bad it would be. If I had known how this would turn out, I would not have put my child through this misery.

Of course, such families are distinctly in the minority. And they may well have been told years before that their child might never learn to walk, talk, or play. But these words are like daggers to the heart of any doctor. Some may have, even perhaps subconsciously, chosen to paint a very bleak picture and be happy to be proven wrong, rather than to offer (in their minds) false hope.

Ultimately, except in very limited circumstances, all prognoses are hypotheses, not facts. Physicians must trust that—with their guidance and counsel—patients and families will make the right decisions for themselves. Every child and every parent is indeed different.

We Treat Souls, Not Just Bodies

42

Throughout my medical training, I purposefully avoided talking, let alone even thinking, about religion while in the hospital. It was one child who changed that.

I am a pediatric intensivist, a doctor who takes care of critically ill children. I am also a Christian but have never overtly brought my faith into the hospital. In my mind, I did not want to create any unnecessary affliction by talking about "taboo" religious topics with patients and their families, unless they intentionally brought it up themselves. Something in my heart that still needed reconciliation was how my faith in God and my job as a physician-scientist fit together—a complex relationship between two of the most important pieces of my identity. Ultimately, as a doctor I found confidence in my years of medical education and training, studying evidence-based medicine and understanding the science and pathophysiology of the human body. My faith in God was something subconscious, *very* subconscious. Although I have seen patients' families, friends, and chaplains praying for healing and recovery, I never seriously thought of it as relevant to any of my medical treatment plans; there was definitely a distinct disconnect. I guess I had never truly believed that prayer could bring physical healing. Surprisingly, it was one of my child patients who made me completely rethink how I think about my faith in God and medicine.

I met Aliyah, a sweet 9-year-old girl, on one of my overnight calls during my critical care fellowship. The general pediatrics ward team called a rapid response code for a PICU consult for her. The ward team informed me that she presented with abdominal pain, fatigue, and trouble breathing and was diagnosed with systemic lymphangiomatosis—a rare disease where her lymphatic system was abnormally developed and dilated and there was fluid accumulating all throughout her body, affecting multiple vital organs. The team was worried about her pain and work of breathing. Aliyah is also an orphan, recently placed into foster care. Hence, there is no guardian at her bedside; she is alone with the medical team. She is breathing fast and hard, her oxygen saturation levels are lower than normal despite getting supplemental oxygen via mask, and her heart is racing at 160 beats per minutes—about double what it should be. Despite her extreme discomfort, Aliyah is particularly polite and responds to all my questions thoughtfully. She tells me that she has

© Springer Nature Switzerland AG 2021
A. F. Schrooten, B. P. Markovitz, *Shared Struggles*,
https://doi.org/10.1007/978-3-030-68020-6_42

trouble breathing and that she has ten out of ten pain everywhere. She is already on a cocktail of extremely powerful analgesics, but we have to transfer her to the PICU to put her on continuous infusions of pain medications. Aliyah would remain in the PICU until her death.

After being transferred to the PICU, this sweet and happy child swiftly made friends with all the staff members, especially the nurses, who quickly learned that she is a devout Christian and always needs her Bible next to her bed. I hear through the grapevine that Aliyah finds comfort in praying with some of the Christian nurses. I am glad that she is getting emotional and spiritual support from our staff, but I am more focused on trying to figure out whether she can qualify and be transferred to a Children's Hospital located halfway across the county to receive a specialized treatment for her disease. It would be her only chance at survival. Unfortunately, over the next few weeks, her disease progresses and we find out that she does not qualify for the specialized treatment due to the severity of her disease. Aliyah suffers a respiratory arrest requiring emergent intubation. She accumulates more fluid in her body and vital organs requiring many invasive procedures including a pericardiocentesis, where accumulated excess fluid around the heart is drained. Through all of this, Aliyah remains bright-eyed when she is conscious, even while intubated. She plays with her Silly Putty when she is in a good enough mood and she continues to pray with the nurses.

In the days close to her death, Aliyah's pain worsens severely. She is in extreme pain in all parts of her body almost constantly without relief despite being on the highest doses of multiple analgesics. One of those nights while I was on call in the PICU, I receive a call at 2 am from her nurse informing me that Aliyah is inconsolable from the pain despite getting multiple bolus doses of opioids. I walk into her room and see that she is crying with her fists tightly clenched, unable to scream because she is intubated and dependent on a mechanical ventilator. Her heart rate is 180 beats per minute and her blood pressure is 160/100. I give her multiple bolus doses of analgesia which bring her no relief. I am frustrated and feel helpless, so I stop to take a moment to think and really look at Aliyah, independent of her pain and sickness.

Here is this sweet girl, an orphan without any family to love on her and be with her during this unfathomably painful time. Yet despite her circumstances, she has remained so positive during all of it. How has she remained so joyful? I see her toys and "magic" Silly Putty bottles scattered around her bedside. Then, I see her Bible. I am quickly reminded of her prayer times and I ask Aliyah, who is writhing in pain, if she would like me to pray for her. She nods affirmatively. I hold her hand and pray aloud for a couple of minutes, asking God to give Aliyah peace and healing, and assert that we know God has a great plan for her, and how much God loves this child. Within 2 minutes after the prayer, Aliyah's heart rate and blood pressure normalized and she fell asleep comfortably. I was stunned. I had never seen anything like this before.

There is much more to medicine than we know. As a critical care physician, I often thought about life from a biological, physiological, and humanistic standpoint because I wanted to provide the most empathic care possible. However, this amazing child showed me that there is so much more to caring for a human being, especially one who is critically ill. Aliyah taught me that even within hospital walls, all patients are more than just their physical bodies. There exists a depth to the purpose and meaning of life that cannot be seen, felt, or measured. Deep within every human, there exists their soul. Though there are limits to physical healing from a medical standpoint, what cannot be seen—the soul—is where our hope and our faith are alive, and, albeit often overlooked, it is ultimately what matters most. Now, as an attending physician in the PICU, I very often think about Aliyah, especially when difficult cases arise. I try and take a step back and remember to view each patient and their families wholly and through a soulful and spiritual lens and to love on my patients entirely. We treat souls, not just bodies. Rest in peace, sweet Aliyah.

Parent Commentary

An important component of the care given to patients by the healthcare team, particularly in the hospital setting, is spiritual care. While most medical institutions have a distinct pastoral care team to address this aspect of care, this should not preclude a physician (or any member of the healthcare team) from offering spiritual care to their patient. Certainly, not every family or patient will welcome spiritual care, nor will every physician be comfortable participating in spiritual care. However, when the recognition and connection is there, both patient and physician will sense it and, in those instances, I do not believe it is inappropriate to act on it.

When this physician reached a point in the care of his patient where his actions in the form of medical interventions did not bring her relief, he paused and reflected. He observed his patient as a whole person, not simply as a body with a disease and in pain that could only be managed with scientific knowledge. He gave attention to the factors that contributed to who Aliyah was as a person—her family situation, her personality, and her faith. While this physician always respected the boundary between his faith and his delivery of medical care, the helplessness he felt in that moment along with his powers of observation lead him to cross that boundary. This physician felt a spiritual connection with his patient and he acted on it. The results were healing for the patient and life-changing for the physician.

As the parent of a child who never spoke a word because of a disease that affected his brain, yet who conveyed so much from a place deep within, I have a true understanding and appreciation for this physician's acknowledgment of the existence of the soul. I believe it is the soul that gives our neurologically devastated child a voice, our seriously ill child the strength to pull through the seemingly impossible, and our dying child the ability to find joy. When you cannot find a physical source or scientific explanation—credit the soul. Indeed, there is much more to the human existence than the physical body.

Physician Commentary

Who could not be moved by this story? It stirs our own souls to read about this physician and this child's soul. Although there are aspects to being human that science cannot yet understand, it does not mean they can be ignored, even or perhaps especially by physicians. There are boundaries, however, that need to be respected when it comes to nonmedical aspects of the physician-patient-parent relationship. The cardinal rule that underlies these limitations is that a physician should never impose their own values upon a patient. Those values might relate to religion, politics, economics, and even sports. In this story, there was alignment between the patient and the physician, and he offered to pray for her because presumably he felt comfortable doing so and knew how spiritual the child was. In situations with there is no obvious alignment, however, such offers are outside the usual boundaries of the practice of medicine. Offering to pray for someone who has not expressed any interest in prayer or religion would be a questionable practice and might be seen as imposing one's value system on the patient.

There is another aspect to this connection between physicians and families that is exemplified by religion but pertains to the more worrisome realms of race, gender, ethnicity, and other similar realms. Does the physician who practices the same religion as the patient before her treat this patient differently? Does the physician who harbors disrespect for members of a religion or race treat such patients differently? Even if only on a subconscious level? Implicit or unconscious bias is real and affects the way we treat each other every day. At least with respect to race, some of the significant discrepancies of patient outcomes have been traced to differences in treatment by healthcare professionals.

While this particular story is one of connectedness and faith, we must be cognizant of the potential dark side of making these connections. Physicians are human. Humans respond differently to other humans who look, talk, and behave as they do. There is nothing wrong with making such nonmedical connections as long as they do not create more distance with patients and families who do not align with our individual beliefs or values. In another day and age, this was called favoritism, and there is no place for that in medicine.

Never Give Up

43

"Your six-month-old son has Gaucher's disease. This is a genetic, fast progressing lysosomal storage disease in which the body lacks an important enzyme needed to break down a fatty chemical called glucocerebroside. Without it, children become disabled and are not expected to live past the age of three. It is extremely rare, it is fatal, and it has no cure."

Upon hearing those four confusing sentences I fell into a black hole. That was until I decided that I was going to move mountains for my son, Nixon. Research was the key. Every day I would type "cure for Gaucher's Disease" in the search bar to try and find every doctor I could who was associated with the disease in one way or another. I wanted to find and work with the experts—the doctors who dedicated their lives to studying the disease. Each time I would talk with one doctor, I would receive another name to call. I was in contact with a scientist in Israel working on a cure and with doctors in Europe who were studying the disease. It was through these doctors that my husband and I were put in contact with a doctor in the United States who specialized in doing stem cell transplants on children with rare diseases. After a phone consultation with her, we were on the next flight across the country for a consultation. This doctor had not transplanted a child with Gaucher's disease before, but after a number of tests and evaluations, she felt that Nixon's disease had been caught early enough and that if we were willing to try, so was she. We live in a world today that gives us so many options, we just have to keep looking and be willing to take risks.

When Nixon was 7 months old, we packed up our belongings and moved across the country where Nixon underwent an umbilical cord stem cell transplant at the only hospital that offered him a chance at a cure. The transplant was a success and he showed amazing strength and resiliency throughout the transplant process. However, it was not without some bumps in the road. A stem cell transplant is not easy. It took 7 months, and during those 7 months Nixon underwent chemotherapy, the stem cell transplant, six surgeries, countless MRIs and CT scans, 5 weeks in the Pediatric Intensive Care Unit, being on a ventilator, and needing to be resuscitated. He proved to us that he was the strongest person we know. After those long 7 months in the hospital, we were finally able to return home.

© Springer Nature Switzerland AG 2021
A. F. Schrooten, B. P. Markovitz, *Shared Struggles*,
https://doi.org/10.1007/978-3-030-68020-6_43

We knew that prior to the transplant, the disease had already caused damage to his small body, but Nixon was not ready to give up the fight. The 2 years following the transplant, Nixon's everyday life became more complicated. We now had a "special needs son" and our vocabulary made us sound like we were medical professionals. Our knowledge and expertise was key to Nixon's survival.

We started our new normal in our new world. Prior to the transplant, Nixon experienced muscle spasms and twitched in his sleep. However, it was not until we started weaning him off all his posttransplant medicines that we realized how bad it was. After sending videos to his doctors and going for an EEG, we found out that Nixon was having seizures. He also developed episodes of a movement disorder. These events compromised his breathing and became dangerous. After a particularly rough day of breathing difficulties, we took Nixon to our local emergency department. We were transferred to the Children's Hospital downtown, a hospital that we originally reached out to when Nixon was first diagnosed. We learned during the first couple of years that when most doctors hear "Gaucher's Disease" they run the other way because of the rarity and severity of the disease. Because there is not a cure, they believe nothing can be done, and that was the case for us with this hospital. On the ambulance ride there, I thought to myself, "Maybe they will finally believe in him. Maybe they will see how strong he is, how well his transplant took and that he is worth fighting for. Maybe they will look past the Gaucher's Type 2 stereotype and look at the fact that he is engrafted, has been 100% donor since his very first chimerism test, and he has not made a single Gaucher cell in almost two years."

Did I believe that these new seizures and movements were the result of his disease? No doubt. We always knew that Nixon would be affected by his disease, but he did not come this far for a movement disorder, muscle spasms, or seizures to take his life. We never wanted Nixon to suffer or have a bad quality of life, but we wanted to make sure that we always had all of our options on the table before we made any rash decisions. We paid attention to the signs Nixon gave us, we took one step at a time, and we waited to see what he told us.

We spent over 2 months at Children's Hospital trying to control his fevers and stabilize the seizures and movements. Almost every benzodiazepine and barbiturate they had in the hospital had gone through Nixon's G-tube. The doctors came to a point where they were at a loss. We were in unchartered territory with his disease and they could not figure out how to keep him stable. His list of medications was longer than a grocery list. The PICU and palliative care teams were going to give him a week, and if he did not show drastic improvement, then they wanted us to make some major decisions. They wanted us to meet with members of the hospice care team to help with our decisions. We were given four options on how to let Nixon go peacefully. Essentially, the options involved giving him fatal doses of pain medications through his IV. They asked who we would want in the room with us when it happened, if we wanted pictures with Nixon, footprints, handprints, necklaces, and other memorabilia.

I asked the PICU team caring for him that day about giving him cannabis (CBD) oil. During my never-ending research, I read about many cases where it helped children who had seizures. They told me it was not an option because it was so new and the clinical trials for it were still ongoing. I knew that clinical trials were actually being done at the hospital we were at, but the trial protocol did not include Nixon's type of disease, which is why he could not be part of the trial. I was angry because they were giving him a week to improve and then our only option was to let him go. They were unwilling to try any new ideas. I knew that if I left it up to the doctors we would be taking Nixon's handprints and footprints in a week. I was ready to pull out all the stops and decided to take matters into my own hands. It was my last "Hail Mary" pass and it had to work because if it did not, then we would lose the war—and Nixon—in 7 days.

I found a reputable vendor and ordered CBD oil, which was conveniently shipped directly to us. This was not a decision that we made lightly and is not something we recommend, but it was literally a matter of life or death for Nixon. I started giving the CBD oil to him when no one was in the room. After a few days, his fevers went away. As the doctors saw improvement they became more aggressive with his respiratory management. He went from high-flow oxygen to regular oxygen. After one full week of giving him the CBD oil, Nixon was sitting up in a chair and smiling. The doctors were speechless. During rounds, one of the doctors said to us, "We honestly have no idea what to say or how this happened. You guys just need to consider yourselves lucky." We shrugged our shoulders and said, "It's Nixon, he does what he wants to do." After 2 weeks, Nixon was transferred out of the PICU and eventually discharged home.

We had two more years of making memories with Nixon. He was able to experience the zoo, birthday parties, a baseball game, fishing, carnivals, snow tubing, Disney World, horseback riding, and so much more. Unfortunately, when he was just over four and a half years old, he caught a virus that caused his body to go haywire. His body was so weak from the disease, and he just did not have the reserve to fight off the effects of the virus.

The virus caused an infection which caused blood clots that went to his brain and his heart, which then led to a stroke. As I watched the medical team perform CPR on my son for over a half an hour, I looked around the room at what they were doing to his body. I saw the look in my husband's eyes and the eyes of the nurses we knew and who knew Nixon. I remembered what another mother who lost her child to this disease told me at the beginning of this journey. She said, "You will just know when he is done. I can't explain it, but he will tell you and you will know." I moved next to Nixon, looked at my precious son, and pushed the medical team away from him. My husband and I whispered to Nixon, "it's okay to go."

I never discredited the opinions of the doctors we encountered. Doctors can only tell you what they know. But there is a reason why all parents are given that "parental instinct." As with Nixon's disease, certain medical conditions can be extraordinarily complex. We experienced many doctors unfamiliar with Gaucher's disease who tried to apply their knowledge to Nixon. There were statements made by doctors that still echo through my head to this day. I heard:

"There is no hope."
"This is just disease progression and there is nothing we can do."
"Unfortunately it is what it is. Just enjoy the time that you have."

We repeatedly heard, "You two are a young family and you can have more children."

Nobody wants to hear this from a doctor and, sadly, many parents hear these words and give up the fight. The doctors who know the medicine have to work with the parents who know the child. Every child has to be given the opportunity to write his or her own story. A successful alliance is key. The medical professional must accept the family as part of the team in order to optimize the care and quality of life of the patient.

We never stopped fighting for our son and this fighting strength began to show doctors that his life was worth fighting for. Nixon surprised many of the doctors and nurses who cared for him. He taught us all compassion, strength, and teamwork. To this day, we are still in touch with many of his doctors and it is because we fought for what we believed in. We showed that anything is possible, that life is worth fighting for, and, most importantly, to never, ever give up.

Parent Commentary

When a child has an incurable or progressive disease, parents often sense from the medical team a feeling of "this child is going to die regardless of what we do" or "there is nothing more we can do." They feel that efforts to intervene or look for answers are not aggressively pursued. However, it is absolutely innate for a parent to want their child to live, and they will not stop looking for hope even when their child's doctors have.

When Nixon was first diagnosed, his parents were told there was no hope for a cure, but they did their research and found the only doctor who gave them a chance. When Nixon's seizures could not be controlled with the best known medicines and treatment available, his parents did their research, took a significant risk, and found a medicine that helped. Throughout the 4 years of Nixon's life, his parents never gave up hope that there was something more they could do for him. They adjusted their hopes according to what Nixon showed them. In the beginning, they hoped for a cure and a healthy little boy, but as Nixon's health declined they hoped for Nixon to get well enough to leave the hospital so they could make memories with him— and they made that happen.

When talking with parents, there is a difference between discussing honest and realistic expectations and blocking off any possibility of hope by saying that nothing more can be done. One of the most compassionate questions a physician can ask a parent is "what is your hope for your child?" This is not a one and done question. It is a question that should be asked repeatedly throughout the child's life and progression of their disease. There is always something to hope for.

Parents understand that doctors do not have all the answers. Parents understand doctors have limited time and resources that have to be focused on those patients whose lives can actually be saved or extended based on the available information and treatments that are known. However, when answers and treatments are not readily known, the parents *will* do the research, send the emails, make the phone calls, and think outside the box to save their child's life. In this age of social media and the ability to connect with researchers and parents across the globe, proactive and dedicated parents are leading the way and having a real impact on the discovery of treatments. As Nixon's parents have so profoundly shown us, parents will go to the ends of the earth to have one more day with their child and they will do it at all costs: financial, emotional, and even ethical. Because one more day with their child is one more day they have hope.

Physician Commentary

There has been a long-standing problem with "fatal" diagnoses; they are self-fulfilling prophesies. If the textbooks say something like "all children with this disease will die in the first year of life," for years, physicians and parents have accepted this dogma and, lo and behold, do not do anything to attempt to sustain the child. Prophesy fulfilled. The world is changing, as new methods of treating diseases and new research is being done all the time. Organ and stem cell (bone marrow) transplants, gene therapy, and new medicines, have all at least started to turn the tide in what were uniformly fatal conditions. Sometimes they only buy time, but as with Nixon and his family, that time was worth every minute. Meanwhile, physicians should absolutely keep an open mind as they partner with families to "push the envelope" insofar as possible.

There is, however, a somewhat dark underbelly to this story, as parents go across the country or around the world to seek the best care for their children. The problem is, only some families—families with the means to do so—can undertake these journeys. Not all families are as sophisticated to seek out and find the one hospital 3000 miles away where hope may be offered. Few have the finances to accomplish such missions, as our disjointed "healthcare system" in the United States can rarely be worked to this advantage for every child. The social determinants of the inequities in healthcare are certainly beyond the scope of this commentary or book, but our readers should be cognizant that for every Nixon, there are dozens of other children with the same diagnosis whose stories likely turned out very differently.

Still, there is always reason—and room in our (parents and physicians) hearts and minds—for hope.

The Sliver of Sky

44

His pained, deep brown eyes met mine with curiosity and then drifted to the window where we could see the sliver of Carolina blue sky peeking over the mountains of medical infrastructure. Mid-morning sunbeams cast shadows of the whirring BiPAP machine and slender metal IV pole on the far wall. He lay in bed with a full face mask with a long blue tube draped over his Carolina Panthers jersey and afghan connecting to the BiPAP machine. His eyes found mine again, asking a question.

He looked at my coat—short, indicating I was a medical student, a student doctor, and feeling every bit of an imposter there in the Pediatric Intensive Care Unit (PICU) with all eyes on me. His eyes moved down to my lap. I was seated in my beloved wheeled companion, affectionately known as "the green machine," by that point worn and dented with love, miles, and grit. He looked at my wheelchair with a perplexed expression filled with disbelief and confusion.

His eyes met mine again, asking me something that it seems only the two of us could hear. I was at that moment supposed to be telling a very important story about an adolescent struggling to breathe with muscles that over time had failed him; now fighting an infection and all of the medical measures our team was proposing for him. I continued, "From a respiratory standpoint: Bi-phasic applied pressure of 28/6, FiO_2 of 28%, we needed to increase the pressure overnight several times."

Outwardly, I looked like a composed fourth year medical student on her acting internship presenting a new admission, auditioning for the part she always wanted, to be a pediatrician. Inwardly, I was playing a familiar part in this drama in the round, the role of a fellow patient sitting in the waiting room, waiting. I held his gaze in answer to his question, "Yes. I know I'm both."

For a moment, no one else was there. We were two people living in bodies that did not play by the rules and that I was so carefully trying to memorize and study. We had never met but regarded each other as companions, we knew very little about each other and yet we knew much. We knew about scars, bullies, beeps in the night, waking up from dreamless, timeless sleep, the wind in our hair flying down a hill on wheels, looking at the sky. Yet we also knew of the endless afternoons, craning our heads tethered to a hospital bed, looking at a sliver of sky aching for just a bit more.

© Springer Nature Switzerland AG 2021
A. F. Schrooten, B. P. Markovitz, *Shared Struggles*,
https://doi.org/10.1007/978-3-030-68020-6_44

"From an electrolyte standpoint ..." I droned on from the script in my hand. He looked again toward the window and back to my wheels and then back to my face and smiled briefly. Then his face changed, suddenly the utter exhaustion and resigned anxiety filled his eyes. His breaths were more labored than when I first examined him a few hours before rounds. I finished my carefully composed monologue in the round in my external voice. I held his gaze as I finished, but he looked away back toward the window, back toward the piercing blue sky that no one else seemed to notice.

The team shifted and so did the moment. The attending intensivist nodded to me as he walked over to examine the patient, the nurse left the circle to talk to the parents who were huddled in the far corner of the room. I stayed in place for a moment feeling as if there were things left unsaid but not sure who was supposed to say them.

The attending whispered to me as I rolled out of the room and down the hall that our patient had lost two brothers a few years back, same disease, and same hospital and that his parents did not want anyone to talk to him about his wishes right now. I looked back down the hall through the plexiglass door. He saw me and our eyes met again, fearful, tired. I nodded; he held my gaze and then looked back to the window. I turned back toward rounds and around the corner told the attending, "Don't you think he already knows?" He looked at me, slightly taken back. I blushed, feeling I had crossed an unseen line.

My day went on, a busy call day that merged into a busy call night, pneumonia, sepsis, asthma, teaching and charting, rolling from the ED to the floor, and back again. My patient in the PICU was stable all day. I visited several times and found him unchanged, sleeping intermittently, his eyelids fluttered when my stethoscope listened to his rattled breathing, and his lips curled in a half smile of acknowledgment. In the wee hours of the morning, my pager squealed and suddenly the senior resident and I flew down the hall. I was grateful for the advantage of wheels as we sped faster and faster.

His distress was audible from the door, beeping monitors, the BiPAP alarming as our team descended to examine and poke and prod. He did not stir. His parents stood in the corner silent, looking anxious, and exhausted. The intensivist came, gestured to the parents and me to the hallway and down the hall to a room with terrible coffee in Styrofoam cups and a cramped table and chairs for conversations such as these.

"Severe acute on chronic respiratory acidosis and respiratory failure in the setting of bilateral worsening pneumonia in advanced neuromuscular disease," the attending listed the litany of diagnoses. The parents sat huddled in the corner holding cups of coffee and staring past the speaker. The attending trailed off and the little room was silent. Finally, the father holding on to his wife's hand, face already hard with grief and with tears glistening at the corners of his eyes, "We've been here before, it's hard for us but our son does not want to suffer as his brothers did, no tubes, no airways."

The attending nodded quickly and quietly called the nurse to transfer the patient to a palliative care suite. I sat in the hard plastic chair, pushed the flimsy box of tissues toward the silently weeping parents, no words seemed enough. As a young doctor, it was so hard to not want to scream, "but WAIT... we could do this...or that," uncomfortable with letting go of our fragile, valiant attempts at holding back the tide. As a fellow person in the waiting room, I found myself profoundly sad, yet equally grateful his suffering would not be prolonged. Grateful for brave parents who quietly advocated and honored him even when I had doubted. Grateful that when so much had been taken from him, he was honored with the power of choice.

The night went on, tiptoes, whispers replaced the beeping and the whirring of the ICU. I found myself startled as the room warmed with a new glow. Until that moment I had not noticed the large windows facing the bed. They showed far more than a sliver of the expansive, lavender-blue sky that glowed with the faintest glare of dawn. As the attending whispered the raw, certain words of "time of death" there were tears, words of gratitude, and a hug I did not feel I deserved. The long night and journey for my patient and his parents ended.

My journey to the other side was paradoxically just beginning. As I wheeled outside a few hours later, it was a beautiful summer morning. I took a long deep, unlabored breath, before flying down the hill, keeping my eyes on the unlimited blue sky, making a silent promise to remember the important teaching, and feeling the bittersweet joy of knowing somehow, he heard our conversation.

He was my first pediatric patient death as a student doctor. Looking back a decade later, I learned much from him. I learned how hard it is for doctors, parents, and caregivers of all roles to let go and honor patients' choices and hopes. About how important it is to listen…really listen to what our patients are telling us. Last, he taught me much about a power I did not know I had. Not just the power of representation of a different perspective in medicine but of empathy and solidarity. Each day I carry these lessons with me still as I enter hospital rooms of sick children and worried parents, teach students and residents, and continue alongside them to learn to be a better listener.

"Hope and lament are twin sisters, walking hand-in-hand." – Emmanuel Katotongue

Parent Commentary

This story shares the unique perspective of a doctor-patient. As a parent, it is also a powerful reminder that our children who live with a life-limiting and/or terminal condition know when their body is failing; they know when they have had enough of the poking, the prodding, and the pain. Our child lets us know what they want and need, whether through their words, or, for our nonverbal child, through their body language. As difficult as it is, we must listen to what they are telling us. The patient in this story was able to articulate his wishes, and while it does not make it any less difficult for a parent to let their child go, I can imagine that hearing your child give you permission to say "no" to further intervention would ease some of the guilt a parent inevitably feels. This patient's parents also had the unusual (and devastating) perspective of having been in this situation before. They knew the consequences of their decisions, as did their son.

While I would never suggest that it is ever comfortable or routine for a physician to advise stopping or withholding treatment, physicians do have the benefit of experiencing what end of life can look like for their patient when "everything" medically possible to stay the inevitable is done versus the compassionate withdrawal or withholding of treatment. Physicians honor their patient's choices looking through a different lens than a parent. As a young medical student, the physician in this story did not yet have the experience of witnessing varied end of life scenarios like a more seasoned physician does; she also had the shared experience with her patient as a person with a disability who had spent time in a hospital as a patient. Her mixed emotions of conflict and gratitude surrounding the death of her patient are understandable. Yet, she came away from the experience recognizing the importance of honoring a patient's choices as both a physician and a patient.

It is exceptionally difficult as a parent to do "nothing" for our child when we have spent our child's entire life doing everything in our power to keep them alive and here with us. We have said yes to the very treatments and technology we are often asked to discontinue at the end of life. How can we possibly do this? I am reminded of what my son's neurologist told me at the end of his life, she told me that by withdrawing and limiting intervention I was not doing nothing, I was just doing things differently.

As the parents and physician in this story show us, and as my son's wise neurologist reminded me, to love your child (and honor your patient) enough to *do things differently* can be the most selfless (and painful) act of love we can give our child (and patient).

Physician Commentary

This is an elegantly written depiction of the impact of a teenager's death had on a physician-in-training. That this student had also spent time in the hospital as a patient seemed to give her an ability to bond, nonverbally, with this child. She heard what he was saying, and he was only talking with his eyes. Physicians must learn to read their patients. I believe I can see despair, fear, pain, exhaustion, and maybe optimism. I could not have read this patient as this medical student was doing. She spoke of a power she did not know she had. This is a rare gift.

The message that we must listen to our patients is a bedrock of creating the patient-physician therapeutic relationship and does not need special powers or gifts. Listening is, however, often easier said than done in pediatrics. Clearly, with infants, toddlers, and even children who are early school-age, we entrust the parents to speak for their children. What is the role of the voice of the older child and especially teenagers? It seems that chronic and complex illnesses can add wisdom to these patients, yet they may also be treading on the road to independent thinking and even rebellion that all children and teens face during maturation. When children and parents disagree on a medical plan, or when parents themselves disagree, particularly when decisions about limiting life-sustaining therapies are at stake, the simple clarity of "listen to your patient" is anything but clear.

This story, however, offers remarkable clarity, as the patient and parents, sadly having gone through this before with two other children, were on the same page with respect to their choice to limit invasive interventions. This young doctor-in-training was presented with a painful but compassionate situation, and she had the special gift to "hear" the message directly from her patient without the need for words.

The Many Voices of Hope

45

I keenly felt the frustration I created during each encounter with the airway nurses and the surgeon's rounding staff. Repeated comments including: "He doesn't come to patient rooms." "You can talk to him in the induction room before surgery tomorrow." "I have never seen him come to the floor." Some comments were meant as reassurances. Others seemed to be sheer exasperation. I held my ground knowing that I could not sign another surgical consent for my daughter without having a real conversation with her surgeon.

Just 3 weeks before, Dani had been released from the hospital to the Ronald McDonald House in anticipation of heading back to our home, 2500 miles away. Everyone was amazed at how well she sailed through recovery after a major airway surgery that resulted in her finally getting her trach out. Dani had been trached since a few days after she was born due to severe airway anomalies. She had three surgical repair attempts with a highly credentialed, local pediatric ENT surgeon by the time she was 3 years old. When the last surgery failed, we decided to make the trip to a world-renowned surgeon across the country to give her the best chance at a healthy life.

The trach was manageable. Dani did not know any different; it was just a part of her. She was used to being connected to an apnea monitor when she went to sleep. She learned to walk around the thick, blue corrugated tubing she was attached to 90% of the time to make sure she had enough humidity getting to her lungs. She had even recently started suctioning her own trach, which kept her lungs clear and her trach plug free. However, we both hated trach changes ever since a traumatic experience where her airway collapsed when we tried to put a new trach in, which resulted in a lot of bleeding and a scary ambulance ride.

She picked up sign language like a champ, having a 400-word vocabulary by the time she was three. Even though she could hear, her cousins, grandparents, aunts, and uncles learned some basic sign language so she could talk to them and not rely on me to interpret everything she wanted to tell them. She was a thriving, happy, and engaged kid living with a complex and life-threatening condition. Of course, we wanted more for her, and we were willing to do what we could to give her a safe

© Springer Nature Switzerland AG 2021
A. F. Schrooten, B. P. Markovitz, *Shared Struggles*,
https://doi.org/10.1007/978-3-030-68020-6_45

airway and healthier life. We wanted her to be able to speak, because even at a young age it was clear she had some extraordinarily strong opinions. We wanted her to be able to participate in school plays and sing in the choir. We wanted her to know that we did everything we could to reduce her limitations in life.

The first week after surgery went great. We met several other "airway" families at the Ronald McDonald House who, like us, had traveled thousands of miles to see the same "Airway Guru," who was viewed as the surgeon of "hope" after everything that could be done by the local ENT had been tried and failed. After the first week, however, Dani began tiring quickly when she would play, and she needed more and more sleep. She started having trouble walking to the playground and we had to revert to taking the elevator rather than climbing one flight of stairs. Something was not right. We had several phone conversations with the airway team and finally went to clinic for an evaluation. The nurse practitioner suggested Dani was probably developing allergies to the local pollen and gave her an inhaler prescription and recommended a daily allergy pill. Over the next several days, Dani continued to decline. I would report in daily with the nurse practitioner, and the staff reluctantly scheduled another scope the following week. I felt like the nursing staff discounted my concerns as those of an overly anxious parent. We tried waiting it out as best we could; however, when Dani reached the point where her chest was retracting significantly and her stridor was audible, I took her to the emergency room in the middle of the night.

She was rushed through triage and it was clear she made the residents incredibly nervous. The team put her on oxygen and when her numbers did not improve, the discussion turned to epinephrine. It was obvious the residents had no idea what to do. I learned when Dani was a baby that she followed my cues in a crisis, so I worked hard to always stay calm in scary situations. Seeing the chaos in the room and the stress on the faces of the medical team terrified me and I do not remember ever being so relieved as when the on-call ENT finally arrived and took control of the situation. Dani was readmitted to the hospital and placed on the airway floor. By the following day, her CO_2 levels were so high and her oxygen saturation so low, she was moved to the ICU, put back on CPAP, and ultimately reintubated. After her recent surgery, her endotracheal (ET) tube size was 4.0. When she was reintubated, the doctors had to force a 2.0 ET tube in. During this time, I spoke with the airway fellows, interns, and nurse practitioners. The team conferred with her surgeon and all agreed she had to go back to surgery. The plan was to cut the new scar tissue out, inject steroids into her vocal cords, and put a stent in to prevent further scarring. I agreed this was the right course of treatment, but I still needed to discuss the plan with her surgeon before I would sign the consent. I needed to know he and I were on the same page about his patient and my daughter.

One of the families I met at the Ronald McDonald House had a young daughter in the hospital recovering from airway surgery like Dani. Recovery was not going well and it was unclear whether she could be safely decannulated (have her trach removed). Her parents were staying in their car in the hospital parking lot with their healthy 5-year-old son until a room finally became available at the Ronald McDonald House. The parents were in a desperate situation. The father spoke frequently about his wishes for his daughter. He explained how he told the doctors and nurses in no uncertain terms would he take his daughter home with a trach again. He said the only acceptable outcome was to have her decannulated. He was willing to have oxygen and CPAP, but keeping the trach in was just unacceptable.

It was an incredibly enlightening conversation because it was the first time I really understood how intolerable this could be for some families. I did not fault him one bit for feeling this way. The life they were living was HARD. They had no family support and incredibly limited resources to care for their daughter. They had their other child living in a car in order to be close to their daughter. Their circumstances were completely different from my own. I had no other children to try to split my time and energy with and spent each night in a hotel prior to getting into the Ronald McDonald House with the full support of my family.

Every time I was pressured to sign the consent form before talking to the surgeon, this father's wishes came to my mind. The same surgeon who would be operating on Dani had recently had a heated conversation with this father who told him that a trach was just not an option for his child. I needed to know it was *my* voice in the surgeon's head when he operated on Dani and not this father's. Once the team finally understood that I was not going to relent, the surgeon came to Dani's room, flanked by six other members of his team. I remember laughing a bit at the sight, thinking, "I'm a 5-foot tall woman. Do you really need this many bodyguards?"

To the surgeon's credit, he was incredibly gracious when he spoke with me. I told him that I appreciated him making the trip to Dani's room and I knew this was out of the ordinary for him. I went on to explain that I had no doubt of his surgical ability but I needed to know he understood my hope for my daughter when she was able to leave the hospital again. Even though we traveled across the country to see him with the hope of getting Dani's trach removed, my ultimate hope for Dani was the best quality of life possible, and for her to be able to participate in life to her own maximum ability, whether that included a trach or not. I was concerned that if he went into surgery believing my biggest hope was to have her decannulated, he might make a less conservative decision about re-traching her. I needed him to know being re-trached was not defeat. If, during surgery, he felt a trach was the safest and best option that would let her get back to running around and playing, then that was the choice I wanted him to make.

He listened intently to everything I had to say. He let me know his preference was always to err on the side of caution. He said, of course his goal was to decannulate, but never at the risk of a child's health or general well-being. He would make the decision based on how best she could thrive, rather than if she could safely survive without a trach. The entire conversation took less than 5 minutes. I appreciated that he spoke directly to me and did not let his "bodyguards" interject when they tried. Once I knew he understood what my hopes were going into this second surgery, I was ready to sign the consent with no reservation. We were on the same page. He listened and I felt heard.

The next day, Dani came out of surgery with a stent and another trach. Her surgeon said he may have been able to avoid another trach, but it would have made recovery harder. I often wonder if Dani would have come out of this second surgery without a trach if I had not been able to have the conversation with the surgeon that I had to fight so hard to get. With her trach back, Dani's energy level came back quickly. Once her airway stabilized, we were allowed to go back to our hometown to wait out the rest of her recovery. She celebrated her fifth birthday with friends jumping in a bouncy castle in the backyard. Two weeks later we made a return trip to see the surgeon again and, this time, Dani was successfully decannulated.

Dani forever changed my understanding of hope. Everyone needs hope, but everyone's hopes are different. For families of children with disabilities and complex chronic conditions, our hopes change as we move through our child's medical journey. We should never assume our hopes align with the hopes of other families or even the hopes—or expectations—of the physicians caring for our child. Once I understood every family, every situation, and every physician may have a different definition of hope, I knew I could not expect Dani's surgeon to know what my hope was. He needed to hear it from me. And I am grateful he listened to me and honored my hopes for my daughter, even as they changed over the course of the time he cared for her.

Parent Commentary

As this story shows us, every family is unique and their hopes are different. That is why it is so important for parents to communicate their hopes to the person they are relying on to help them and their child achieve those results (in this case, the child's surgeon.) Without effective communication, assumptions can be made. It would have been reasonable for the surgeon in this story to assume that Dani's mother would only be happy if her daughter returned home without a trach—after all, they traveled 2500 miles because that was their hope. Certainly, the surgeon would never place the hopes of the parent over their child's safety; however, he cannot help but be influenced by what he hears from the parents who bring their children to him as their last hope. In fact, it sounds like the surgeon would have considered a different course if this parent had not had the conversation with him that she had to push so hard to get.

The parent in this story was exceptionally assertive and a strong advocate for her daughter in communicating what she wanted going into the second surgery. However, from my own experience as the parent of a child with a rare and complex condition that could not easily be "fixed," I also think that parents can sometimes be reluctant to express what their hopes are because we cannot bear to hear that what we want for our child is not possible. This is why I believe it is just as important for doctors to ask parents, "what do you hope for?" and regularly ask this question as the child's course changes or disease progresses. Someone has to initiate the conversation, and if the parents are not able to, then the physician should take the lead. Physicians can open the lines of communication and help parents identify their hopes, and together they can navigate the child's ever-changing course.

As a good friend of mine says, "hope is a funny thing." And it truly is. Hope is what drives us to be relentless advocates, yet hope also slows us down by forcing us to reflect on and appreciate what is most important. When our child is born with a rare disorder or complex medical condition, we hang on to the hope of giving our child as "normal" a life as possible and we set the bar and expectations high. We push hard for what we want. However, hope is not static; time and circumstances shift our focus. Our hopes become less about measurable progress and more about wanting our child to feel safe and loved; wanting them to not be in pain; and wanting to have them with us for as long as possible. Like Dani's mother, we adjust our hopes when we have to, because our child's life is what matters most.

Physician Commentary

Creating a shared mental model between physicians and parents is essential to cement the bonds of trust necessary for a therapeutic relationship. Part of that mental model is expectations, or hopes. As much as it is in the parent's hands to be clear about what they hope for, it is the physician who—after thoroughly understanding the parent's position— has to frame the boundaries of expectations. I was struck by the expectations of the father of another patient that stated "the only acceptable outcome was to have her decannulated." Frankly, painting a physician into a corner like this does nothing to engender trust and open communications. In fairness, maybe this father did not state his wishes to the surgeon so defiantly, and the struggles this family was enduring at the time were truly very distressing. For most medical conditions though, there simply cannot be only one acceptable outcome.

Honest expressions of hopes and wishes, impressing upon the physician the values you hold for your child are critical. Physicians need to listen deeply to these expressions and seek them out themselves if not spontaneously offered by families.

Mothers Club

46

I could always tell when Sara was admitted. There were mustache stickers on all the pictures adorning the walls of the Pediatric Intensive Care Unit (PICU). Something with a hula skirt and a coconut dangled from the Nurse Director's office. These were my first clues that a VIP—very important patient—was in the house. Her mother, Rei, would decorate the unit when they were admitted during the wee hours of the morning. It is not that every patient is not important, but Sara was different.

Sara was born with a chromosomal abnormality that most of us read about in textbooks but had never seen in a patient living into adolescence. Sara's trisomy 16 mosaicism conferred upon her developmental delays, seizures, and heart disease. Her parents conferred upon her love, grace, humor, and dignity. For her medical team, there were three truths in caring for Sara: (i) always ask for the updated five-page manifesto her mother, Rei, carried with her; (ii) always check in with her private pediatrician—an exemplary human being who built into his practice the care of a dozen technologically dependent and chronically medically complex patients and was always Sara's advocate; and (iii) include Rei in every conversation and listen well. Rei carried in the deep recesses of her brain the "history of Sara." She could describe every event that could not be medically explained and list the theories we gave for the medical condition we were presented with. In truth, there were no medical books that could describe the physiology we experienced with Sara.

―――――

Rei As a parent, when you are planning a family, having a medically complex child is not something we think about. We think about ballet classes, sleep overs, soccer, first days of school, dress up, dresses, and frilly bows. Having a child that would defy odds was not in the picture. We had no idea that Sara would need open heart bypass surgery at 2 days old. We did not know she would have a cleft palate. We did not know she would need a feeding tube. We did not know she would have seizures. We did not know anything about the journey we were about to embark on. The first few days in the NICU to the PICU for recovery from open heart surgery were

© Springer Nature Switzerland AG 2021
A. F. Schrooten, B. P. Markovitz, *Shared Struggles*,
https://doi.org/10.1007/978-3-030-68020-6_46

overwhelming. It was then that I started to mourn the death of having a normal child. Those dreams I had were gone in the blink of an eye, just like that. I was devastated, but I was also overjoyed with a brand new baby.

––––––

I never knew the "healthy" Sara, - but I knew too well the critically ill Sara. Aware of her surroundings, but not always able to communicate with us, Sara wore a bell on her wrist to let us know she wanted something when she was well enough to communicate. Sara delighted in tinfoil and the sensation and sound of crumpling it. She was cared for by a team of home nurses and her parents in the family living room that was converted into her bedroom. Her older brother went through all the stages of childhood and adolescence with a sense of how special his sister was and the reality that some mornings he would wake up and Sara and Rei had left in the middle of the night to be admitted to the hospital. Sara's visits to the PICU were becoming more frequent and lasting longer. More often than before, we could not explain all the phenomena that she presented with. All the while, Rei would be at her bedside taking care of Sara and educating the next generation of pediatric residents rotating through the PICU on the nuances of caring for a child with a complex medical condition.

––––––

Rei   Sara had a way about her. She was fiercely independent and yet needed help with all of her daily activities. She was naughty and sassy. She had an extremely wicked sense of humor and thought any sort of fall or injury to her caregivers was hysterical. She would laugh and smirk at us. She did not communicate in a conventional way. Before being placed on a ventilator and having a tracheostomy she knew two words, "no" and "mama." After the transition to a ventilator she learned new ways to communicate with us. She would shake her head vigorously. If things were going to happen, it was her way or no way. She could give you one look or an eye roll and you knew she meant business.

I firmly believe that Sara was here to teach. She taught a group of people to become a team of providers. We never made a move until everyone discussed the pros and cons of treatments. Rounds at the bedside were more of a brainstorming session. I gained my PhD in Sara. Residents were eager to try new treatments or suggestions. I had been burned by residents one too many times and was always hesitant. I knew the schedule of lab draws and testing procedures. I knew if a resident came unprepared to rounds. One of our team nurses once asked for Tylenol and the resident responded with "No." I let this go on for a few minutes and then I got up from where I was sitting and leaned over my daughter and the hospital bed with my hands firmly planted on the bedrail. I looked this resident in the eye and gave him an earful. I told him that Sara can be a very scary kid. She does not take days to let you know she is sick. When she gets sick she does it in a matter of hours. She spirals out of control and then we are chasing her. Her nurse today is one of her team nurses that has followed us and has seen Sara at her sickest and you have not seen what this child is capable of. If she asks for Tylenol you write the order for Tylenol. You are new to this team and if you fall behind the eight ball I will become THAT mom. You do not want to see me come unhinged over Tylenol, so if the nurse says she thinks Sara needs Tylenol and things are not adding up, get your orders into the computer now. Pull all the labs you need and start getting a plan together. I guarantee that if Sara is going septic she will be on fluids, TPN, and antibiotics by tomorrow, so do not make me ask you for Tylenol.

So, yes, I called a few residents out. In my chaotic world of Sara, there were few things I had control of, but the things I had control of I did fiercely. I needed to know that the people learning and treating Sara knew that she did not follow a textbook. Whatever you read did not apply to my girl. The attendings and I had conversations about treatments and plans. We needed to be a team and all learn from Sara. I was the expert in Sara-isms and I had to effectively communicate to the team what was going on and try to stay two steps ahead of Sara.

––––––

The night - Sara died I was on-call. Sara's cardiac rhythm began to change, the intervals between her heart beats extended too long between each beat and it was not long before the heart that had outpaced its expectancy by a decade broke. While I remember the conversation that night with Sara's family, it was the celebration of Sara's life that took place a few weeks later that I will never forget. In the midst of their grief, her parents turned to all of us to remember and celebrate the little girl who defied the odds. With mustache stickers around the room, they helped us heal and close the chapter on a very special time we shared caring for Sara. Newly minted members of the club of parents who have survived a child's death, her parents were moving forward and planning how they could now give back to those who never had a chance to prepare for the end of their child's life, for those for whom death had come far too early and far too unexpectedly.

––––––

Rei   The night Sara passed Leah was on service. I got the call from Dan to come quickly as Sara had coded. I quickly got into my car, in my pajamas, and drove as fast as I could to the hospital. I pulled into the entryway, almost leaving the van running as I ran up to the front desk. I had a fight with the security guard about taking me up in the code elevators. The elevators I knew existed because I was involved with the hospital on so many committees. The security guard told me that he could not because they did not have those elevators. I explained to him that my daughter was upstairs coding and that I needed to get up there, now. It was then that my phone rang and Dan asked where I was. I tried to tell him, and then Leah got on the phone. She told me she was sending nurses down to get me. The security guard finally took me up the elevator. When he saw the nurses standing in a line waiting for their turn to do chest compressions, he left. I walked into a sea of faces, all of them there for Sara, waiting for their turn. I asked them to please stop. Those were the hardest but most peaceful words I could say at that moment. My girl was done and I needed to let her go peacefully. I crawled into bed with her and held her and sobbed.

In that moment my life once again forever changed. I lost my little girl. The love of my life. The reason I got up and fought so fiercely every day. My body went numb and the tears flowed. They flowed for the loss of my Sara and the loss of my life as I knew it. I bathed her for the last time that night. Rolling her over to feel the warmth still coming from her body. Bathing her with my best friend who rushed to be with me in those moments. Having her reassure me that Sara looked beautiful as she did her hair for the final time. Everything was final in that room at that moment. My friends and family gathered. We let Sara go, saying our goodbyes thinking about what we would do with her body. The thought of putting her in the ground was too heartbreaking for me, for her to be alone and for me not to be able to see her. We made the decision to have her cremated so that I could keep her close where I needed her.

In the months since Sara passed, I am living my new normal in a house that was once a bustle of activity with nurses in and out of our home, alarms going off, and phone calls to doctors and the insurance company. The quiet echo of a house now devoid of medical equipment and supplies. My body now showing the signs of 12 years of hard work, stress, and sleep deprivation. Would I change things? Not a chance. I am now living the life of a too soon empty nester. My husband and I, partying like we are in college but in the bodies of 40-year-olds. This too is hard, but Sara would have wanted it this way. For us to have fun and experience life. To fight for the underdog and to keep teaching what she taught us. I am always asked how we did it and how we are doing it now. Our motto then and still today is: you never know what is going to happen tomorrow and you do not get a second chance at today. So live life to its fullest. Make good choices. Have a drink or three. Have fun and do good things.

―――――

I had - lunch the other day with a friend I have known for more than 20 years, and who every year takes on a more powerful meaning for me. We met in the 1990s and what started off as an acquaintance has grown over the years into this very special friendship. We share a history of taking care of her son. Along the way we shared his transition from a healthy baby to a critically ill baby to a technologically complex boy to a chronically ill teenager. At our most recent visit, as we dined on salads and lemon tarts, my friend shared with me that she was in town to spend the weekend with a very solemn club she avoided being comforted by—mothers of children who had died. Our friendship has grown out of my first being her son's doctor and later being her confidante.

After we finished our lunch and said goodbye, I wondered what her weekend would be like. It had been more than 3 years since her son died and only now was she ready to make this journey. To meet in a room and talk with other mothers about the raw loss they experienced, the grief that never goes away, and the impact of their child's death on their other children and their spouses. The participants were meeting at a central location at the airport to catch a bus to take them to the retreat location for the weekend. How would they identify each other at the airport, I wondered? What do you say when you walk past each other in the aisle of the bus knowing that the women on the right of you and to the left of you have shared your greatest loss: the death of your child? What common spirit do they all share to be so resilient and caring that allows them to come together to help each other heal? What is their focus that helps them get out of bed every day and start anew?

The number of mothers that are members of this club that I now call friends is growing. Perhaps this is a reflection of how long I have been practicing or the connections I continue to make with families who share their children with me. Perhaps it is our advancements in medicine that allows more fragile children to live past infancy only to die in my unit. When I was much younger I rejoiced in being an inpatient provider and never having a clinic practice. Every patient was new, every family was unique, and every experience had a beginning and an end. As I have matured as a pediatric critical care medicine physician, I have discovered that in fact I do have a group of patients I follow on a regular basis. I have built a strange private practice. There are a group of children I follow, see their parents a few times a year for a PICU admission and along the way watch their children grow up. These special children have made me a better doctor and person over the years. They have taught me to listen better and to partner with their parents—true experts in their child's conditions–in a way I never imagined I would. These children and their families have taught me how to celebrate life.

The mothers I know well who belong to this club have all gone on to make a difference and change the world. One left teaching to become a nurse. One established a respite program for families with chronically ill children. One is building a camp for children with disabilities and has adopted a child with the same disabilities as her daughter who died had. One is building a foundation to help support families of children with chronic illness. As I wonder what the world will look like in another decade or two, where glaciers will be and who will be guarding nuclear missiles, these families tell me that as long as we take care of each other, there is still hope. These mothers have made me a better person by teaching me the true meaning of caring and respect, love and grace, humor and dignity.

Parent Commentary

As Sara's mother shares, few of us ever envisioned being the parent of a medically fragile and complex child when we thought about our life with children. Many of us likely had never seen the inside of a Children's Hospital or Pediatric Intensive Care Unit before our child was born. But we quickly gained the knowledge and confidence we needed to become a fierce advocate for our child. We are the one constant in our child's life and with each hospital admission and each encounter with a new doctor, we stand ready to take the lead because we know our uniquely complex child best.

The hospital becomes a second home, whether we are spending time in clinic or find ourselves inpatient because, despite our best efforts, we are unable to manage our child's precarious health at home. As we settle into yet another inpatient admission, there is nothing more comforting than seeing the familiar face of your favorite attending—the one who knows you and your child well and who greets you with a smile and hug. There is an incredible sense of relief knowing that the degree of advocating that will be required of you this admission will be greatly reduced because this doctor will be *your* frontline advocate. She will let the team know that you are an experienced parent who should be listened to. Because we often see more of our child's doctors than we do our own friends, we cannot help but become attached to these special people who care for our children. They see us at our worst—sleep deprived and disheveled—and they see us at our best, standing guard at our child's bedside ready to take on the world (or the resident who risks questioning us).

As our children become older and somewhat more stable, many of us feel called to take what we have learned as medical parents, advocates, and as members of a close-knit community and do what we can to help others who are similarly situated. Our children change us in profound ways, whether we are called to advocate for one or for many. Our children also introduce us to the most remarkable individuals who devote their lives to caring for the most fragile children. And if we are really fortunate, we have the privilege of connecting with that one doctor who advocates for us, thinks about us, worries about us, finds hope in us, and calls us "friend."

Physician Commentary

Throughout this book, we have heard from parents and physicians, but now we hear from both, in one story about the little girl named Sara. In many ways, this joint story confirms the lessons from this book. The parents of these children know them really, really well. Not just their medical history, but their spirit and unique methods of communicating. These parents are always asked to walk a fine line between showing a modicum of respect for the physicians yet advocating for their child when they truly know more about them than the doctors. As we can see here, some parents will not hesitate to speak up forcefully when it is needed. Ironically, if a senior physician were to speak to a trainee with the language that Rei uses with the resident in the Tylenol episode, the senior physician would be ostracized for highly unprofessional behavior. (So parents, please try your best to be nice to our trainees—they are still learning and can be easily bruised!)

And once again, we learn the impact of these complicated children and their loving parents on a physician and how these interactions can open one's eyes, ears, minds, and hearts in truly meaningful ways. Ultimately, despite all our scientific advancements, learning medicine remains an apprenticeship. We certainly do not learn how to manage complex patients like Sara in medical school and are barely able to absorb lessons as deep as these during training. It can take years of practice, listening, and finally learning to become the type of physician that is highlighted in this book as a true and trusted partner. I do not think it to be unintentional when we say we are "practicing" medicine. Few of us ever really get it right and need to keep practicing, day in and day out. When we have parent partners as highlighted in this book, practice can make perfect for these most complicated and vulnerable children.

Glossary

Acute conditions that are severe and sudden in onset.

Attending an attending physician is a physician who has completed residency and practices medicine in their chosen specialty. An attending physician typically supervises fellows, residents, medical students, and other practitioners.

BiPAP stands for bilevel positive airway pressure. A BiPAP machine provides breathing support with pressurized air delivered through a face mask or nasal mask. A higher amount of air pressure is delivered when you breathe in.

Bronchoscopy a procedure that allows your doctor to examine your lungs and air passages.

Broviac a special intravenous line that is inserted under the skin on the chest that allows for long-term access to the blood.

Chronic conditions or diseases that are persistent or otherwise long-lasting in their effects.

CPAP stands for continuous positive airway pressure. A CPAP machine delivers the same amount of pressurized air as you breathe in and out and is usually delivered through a face mask or nasal mask.

Decannulated the removal of a tracheostomy tube.

Desatting to undergo a decrease in the oxygen saturation level in the hemoglobin.

Endotracheal (ET) tube a flexible plastic tube that is placed through the mouth into the trachea and connected to a ventilator to help a patient breathe.

ENT a doctor who specializes in diagnosing and treating the diseases of the ears, nose, and throat. Also called an otolaryngologist.

Extracorporeal membrane oxygenation (ECMO) a life support machine that replaces the function of the heart and lungs.

Extubated the removal of an endotracheal tube (ETT) from a patient's airway.

Fellow a physician who has completed their residency and elects to complete further training in a specialty. The fellow is a fully credentialed physician who chooses to pursue additional training in a subspecialty.

Gastrostomy tube (G-tube) a tube inserted through the abdomen that delivers nutrition directly to the stomach.

Gestational age the common term used during pregnancy to describe how far along the pregnancy is.

© Springer Nature Switzerland AG 2021
A. F. Schrooten, B. P. Markovitz, *Shared Struggles*,
https://doi.org/10.1007/978-3-030-68020-6

GI doctor a gastroenterologist. A doctor who is an expert in digestive health and issues related to the stomach, intestines, bowels, and also a number of other organs related to the entire digestive tract.

Intubated the insertion of an endotracheal tube into the airway for mechanical ventilation.

Multidisciplinary consists of several healthcare professionals from differing disciplines working together to provide the highest quality of care for their patients.

Pediatric hospitalist pediatricians who specialize in the care of hospitalized children.

Pediatric intensivist pediatricians who specialize in the care of critically ill children who are hospitalized in the Pediatric Intensive Care Unit.

Resident a doctor in training who has graduated medical school. Residency can range from an additional 2 years of education to an additional 7 years of training, depending on the specialty. In the first year of training, residents are sometimes called interns.

Tracheostomy (trach) a hole that surgeons make through the front of the neck and into the windpipe (trachea). A tracheostomy tube is placed in the hole to keep it open for breathing.

Index

A

Advance care planning, 145
Advanced Practice Registered Nurse (APRN), 210, 211
Advocacy, 157–160
    parent commentary, 159, 160
    physician commentary, 160
Agency for healthcare research and quality (AHRQ), 174
Airway obstruction, 24
Altered path, 83, 84
    parent commentary, 85
    physician commentary, 85, 86
American education system, 141
Arnold's syndrome, 31
Ataxia, 196

B

Bedside strength tests, 14
Best laid plans, 57, 58
    parent commentary, 59
    physician commentary, 60
BiPAP machine, 51, 52
Brain aneurysm and stroke, 91
Brain damage
    ACTH treatment, 224
    communication device, 225
    follow-up appointment, 224
    hope in medicine, 225
    infantile spasms, 224
    internet diagnosis, 223
    movements, 224
    neurology team, 224
    NICU stay, 223
    physicians' attitudes, 226
    pre-judgmental thoughts, 224
    prognosis, 225, 226

C

Cannabis (CBD) oil, 232, 233
Cardiac transplantation, 105
Cardiac unit, 202
Care management, 176
Ceiling- and wall-mounted lift-and-transport system, 174
Cerebellar atrophy, 197
Cerebral palsy, 9
Chiari 2 decompression, 182
Chronic health issues, 119
Chronic respiratory acidosis
    attending intensivist, 238
    BiPAP machine, 237
    doctor-patient perspective, 239, 240
    internship, 237
    medical measures, 237
    palliative care suite, 238, 239
    patients' choices and hopes, 239
    physician-in-training, 240, 241
    PICU, 237
    time of death, 239
    utter exhaustion and resigned anxiety, 238
Chronic respiratory failure, 168–171
Communication and empathy, 200
Compassion and empathy, 199
Compassion in medicine, 23–25
    parent commentary, 25, 26, 29, 30
    physician commentary, 26, 30
Complex care program, 174
"Complex Care" teams, 186
Congenital Central Hypoventilation Syndrome (CCHS), 129
Consistency and communication, 182
Cooling process, 142
Courageous parents network (CPN), 177
critical care physicians, 99

© Springer Nature Switzerland AG 2021
A. F. Schrooten, B. P. Markovitz, *Shared Struggles*,
https://doi.org/10.1007/978-3-030-68020-6

D
Decompression surgery, 183
Defense mechanism, 185
Detached concern, 106
Doctor extended compassion, 29
Doctor-patient relationship, 97
Doctor-patient-friend relationship, 97
"Do Not Resuscitate/Do Not Intubate"
        (DNR/DNI), 36, 212, 215
Dystonia, 147

E
Early Care Hospice Team, 120, 121
Electronic record, 114
End of life care, 122, 154, 165, 215, 216
End-of-life decision, 21, 121, 142–145,
        149, 164
Epilepsy, 9, 196

F
Façade of detachment, 106
Fontan, 52
Frequent flyer, 113, 118
Frustration, 124
Full disclosure, 67–69
    parent commentary, 69, 70
    physician commentary, 70, 71

G
Gastrostomy-jejunostomy (GJ) feeding
        tube, 43–45
Gastrostomy tube (G-tube), 3, 5
Gaucher's disease, 231–234
Gene therapy, 235
Glucocerebroside, 231
The Green Machine, 237
Grueling training, 185

H
Hope in medicine, 189–193, 201, 202, 206
    airway anomalies, 243
    chronic conditions, 246
    communication with parents, 246, 247
    conversation, 245
    decannulation, 245, 246
    disabilities, 246
    endotracheal tube, 244, 245
    nurse practitioner, 244
    parent commentary, 193
    physician commentary, 194

    resources to care, 245
    scary situation, 244
    shared mental model, 247
    sign language, 243, 244
    surgical repair, 243
Hospice care, 122, 148, 149, 164
Hourglass brain, 202
Hydrocephalus, 147
Hyperbolic-sounding breath, 203
Hypotonia, 196

I
If We Are Paying Attention, 61–63
    parent commentary, 64
    physician commentary, 65
Impending doom, 150
India pale ale (IPA), 175
Insufflator-exsufflator, 83
Intellectual disability, 196
Intensive inpatient therapy, 119

K
Ketogenic diet, 87
Kidney stones, 161
Kids like these, 39–41
    parent commentary, 41, 42
    physician commentary, 42
KIF1A-related disorder, 196–198

L
Learning together, 77–80
    parent commentary, 80
    physician commentary, 81
Life-altering and/or life-limiting diagno-
        sis, 89, 90
Life-saving interventions, 135
Life-threatening illness, 205
Listeners, confidants, and consolers, 10
Loss of function and fearing, 203

M
Meaningful interactions, 36
Medical journal, 204
Medically complex child, 205
Medical team and nurse management, 40
Medication decisions, 144
Minute by minute, step by step, 27–29
Movement disorder, 232, 234
MTM-CTM family connection, 177
Muscle biopsy, 15

Muscular Dystrophy Association (MDA), 84
Myeloschisis, 181
Myotubular myopathy (MTM), 152, 153
Myriad of medical experts, 195

N
Neonatal Intensive Care Unit (NICU), 87
Newcomer Parent Night, 141
Noninvasive ventilation trial, 168
Non-verbal children, 117

O
Operating room documenter, 27
Operating team extended compassion, 29
Optic nerve atrophy, 197
Organ transplant, 235

P
Pain management, 162, 185
Palliative care, 121, 122, 154, 155,
    163–165, 183
Palliative care fellowship, 115
Paramedics, 141
Parent decision-making, 13–15
    parent commentary, 16
    physician commentary, 17
Parental intuition, 108
Parenting, 5
Patient-and-family engagement, 178
Patient-family relationship, 173
Patient management, 97
"Patient Relations" teams, 185
Pediatric complex care, 173
Pediatric early care team with hospice, 120
Pediatric Intensive Care Unit (PICU), 13–16,
    217, 237
    advancements in medicine, 253
    apprenticeship, 254
    cardiac rhythm, 251
    care taking, 252
    chromosomal abnormality, 249
    chronically ill children, 253
    code elevators, 251
    continuity physicians, 135
    end of life, 251
    hospital admission, 253, 254
    insurance company, 252
    medically complex child, 249, 250
    resilient and caring, 252
    team of providers, 250, 251
    treatments and plans, 251

Pediatric palliative care
    aggressive care, 218
    critical evaluation, 219
    evidence-based medicine, 219
    experimental stem cell transplant, 217
    gastrostomy tube, 219
    Gaucher disease type 2, 217, 218
    information and guidance, 220
    inpatient settings, 221
    knowledge, experience, and belief, 220
    life-limiting condition, 219
    medical professionals, 220
    neurodevelopmental specialist, 218
    parent advocate, 220
    seizures and abnormal movements,
        217, 218
    tracheostomy, 219
Pediatric palliative care fellowship, 113
Pediatric Physical Medicine and
    Rehabilitation, 201
Perioperative care for children, 175, 177
Peripheral neuropathy, 196
Permanent brain injury, 10
Permission seeking, 31–33
    parent commentary, 33, 34
    physician commentary, 34
Photograph, 73, 74
    parent commentary, 74, 75
    physician commentary, 75
Physician-parent interaction, 206, 207
Physician-patient relationship, 95
Physiologically stressful surgery, 174
Plumbing-type surgeries, 202
Pneumonia, 124
Post-traumatic stress, 92
Pre-operative care, 175
Progressive disease, 234

Q
Quality of life, 35, 37, 121, 232, 234
    APRN, 210, 211
    authority and experience, 213
    autonomic suffering, 212
    brain stem malformation and compres-
        sion, 209
    Chiari decompression, 210
    chronic ventilatory support, 215
    cognitive/physical disabilities, 212
    competence and success rate, 210
    desaturation, 209
    DNR, 212
    dysautonomia, 214
    end-of-life care, 216

Quality of life *(con't)*
    full blown mastitis, 210
    G-tube surgeries, 211
    life-altering decision-making, 214
    medical ethics, 211, 212, 216
    medical, moral and psychological
            companionship, 211
    open sacral spine, 209
    palliative care team, 211, 212, 215
    parental medical decision making, 213
    post-op, 209
    trach surgery, 212
    tracheostomy, 211
    treatment, 213, 214
    urinary catheterization, 212

R
Real-life superhero, 91–93
    parent commentary, 93
    physician commentary, 94
Re-learning to listen, 135–137
    parent commentary, 138
    physician commentary, 138, 139
Residency and fellowship training, 184
Respectful communication, 183
Respiratory virus, 205
Retinopathy of prematurity, 77
Reuniting families, 19–21
    parent commentary, 21
    physician commentary, 22
Risk-benefit ratio, 53
Road map, 123–126
    parent commentary, 126, 127
    physician commentary, 127

S
Sacred relationship, 35–37
    parent commentary, 37, 38
    physician commentary, 38
Seizure rescue medications, 88
Seizures, 232, 234
Septic infection, 119
Shared experience, 101–103
    parent commentary, 103, 104
    physician commentary, 104
Short attention span, 105

"Show & Tell", 152
Shunt revision surgeries, 124
Skin discoloration, 203
Smile worth saving, 43–45
    parent commentary, 46
    physician commentary, 46, 47
Social media, 235
Social skills, 203
Spina bifida, 183
Spinal fusion surgery, 39, 174
Spinal Muscular Atrophy Type 2 (SMA), 83
Spiritual care
    christian nurses, 228
    continuous infusion, 228
    critical care fellowship, 227
    multiple analgesics, 228
    pastoral care team, 229
    peace and healing, 228
    physical healing, 227, 229
    physician-patient-parent relationship, 230
    scientific knowledge, 229
Steep learning curve, 95
Stem cell transplant, 231, 232, 235
Stroke, 202, 204

T
Team harlie, 51–54
    parent commentary, 54, 55
    physician commentary, 55
Teamwork, 129–131
    parent commentary, 132
    physician commentary, 133
Telemedicine, 118
Therapeutic relationship, 98
Tracheostomy surgery, 14
Tumultuous pregnancy, 77

V
Value-laden questions, 109
Vascular ring, 13
Virus, 233

W
Western medical ethics, 22
Whole exome cenetic sequencing, 196